Mickey C. Smith, RPh, PhD

The Rexall Story
A History of Genius and Neglect

*Pre-publication
REVIEWS,
COMMENTARIES,
EVALUATIONS ...*

"**M**ickey Smith has dug deep to uncover an inside look at Rexall, their successes, failures, pundits, and bandits. His book is a surefire bulls-eye in its quest to uncover nostalgia for former Rexallites and their customers. One is left to ask, with a heavy sense of loss, 'How can things go so right for so long only to wither and die in the end?' Was it greed, ego, or simply disinterest that led to Rexall's extinction as America's largest and leading virtual drug chain? Although the Rexall 'family' is gone, Dr. Smith preserves its memory for all the pharmacists, their families, and their customers who viewed the orange and blue Rexall sign as a homecoming of sorts in towns and cities across the American landscape. As hard-hitting as a Rexall One-Cent Sale!"

Dick Hartig, CEO
Hartig (formerly Rexall) Drug Stores

"**H**aving grown up working in my father's Wood Rexall drugstore, literally on the corner of Main Street, I thoroughly enjoyed Smith's chronical of this important part of pharmacy's history. He has captured many voices of the grass roots of pharmacy that went such a long way in shaping our profession and our business in much of the twentieth century. Smith brings the 4-Ps of marketing to life with this very special part of Americana."

Kurt A. Proctor, PhD, RPh
President, National Association of Chain Drug Stores Foundation

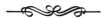

"**D**r. Smith has once again done the profession he loves a tremendous service by capturing this amazing story from our history. The important lessons contained in Rexall are too numerous to fully grasp on first reading. This should be required reading for every public-serving practice in the twenty-first century."

Lucinda Maine, PhD, RPh
Executive Vice President, American Association of Colleges of Pharmacy

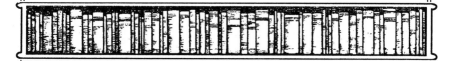

Pharmaceutical Products Press®
An Imprint of The Haworth Press, Inc.
New York • London • Oxford

The Rexall Story
A History of Genius and Neglect

PHARMACEUTICAL PRODUCTS PRESS®
Pharmaceutical Heritage:
Pharmaceutical Care Through History

Mickey C. Smith, PhD
Dennis B. Worthen, PhD
Senior Editors

Laboratory on the Nile: A History of the Wellcome Tropical Research Laboratories by Patrick F. D'Arcy

America's Botanico-Medical Movements: Vox Populi by Alex Berman and Michael A. Flannery

Medicines for the Union Army: The United States Army Laboratories During the Civil War by George Winston Smith

Pharmaceutical Education in the Queen City: 150 Years of Service, 1850-2000 by Michael A. Flannery and Dennis B. Worthen

American Women Pharmacists: Contributions to the Profession by Metta Lou Henderson

A History of Nonprescription Product Regulation by W. Steven Pray

A Social History of Medicines in the Twentieth Century: To Be Taken Three Times a Day by John K. Crellin

Pharmacy in World War II by Dennis B. Worthen

Civil War Pharmacy: A History of Drugs, Drug Supply and Provision, and Therapeutics for the Union and Confederacy by Michael A. Flannery

Federal Drug Control: The Evolution of Policy and Practice edited by Jonathon Erlen and Joseph F. Spillane

Dictionary of Pharmacy edited by Dennis B. Worthen

The Rexall Story: A History of Genius and Neglect by Mickey Smith

The History of American Homeopathy: The Academic Years, 1820-1935 by John. S. Haller Jr.

The Rexall Story
A History of Genius and Neglect

Mickey C. Smith, RPh, PhD

Pharmaceutical Products Press®
An Imprint of The Haworth Press, Inc.
New York • London • Oxford

381.456151 SMITH 2004

Smith, Mickey C.

The Rexall story

Published by

Pharmaceutical Heritage Editions, a series from Pharmaceutical Products Press®, an imprint of The Haworth Press, Inc., 10 Alice Street, Binghamton, NY 13904-1580.

Cover design by Jennifer M. Gaska.

Cover photo used by permission of the Terminal Railroad Association.

Library of Congress Cataloging-in-Publication Data

Smith, Mickey C.
    The Rexall story : a history of genius and neglect / Mickey Smith.
        p.; cm.
    Includes bibliographical references and index.
    ISBN 0-7890-2472-1 (hard : alk. paper)—ISBN 0-7890-2473-X (soft : alk. paper)
    1. Rexall Drug Company—History. 2. United Drug Company—History. 3. United-Rexall Drug, Inc. 4. Rexall Drug and Chemical Company—History. 5. Dart Industries—History. 6. Liggett, Louis, d. 1946. 7. Drugstores—United States—History. I. Title.
    HD9666.9.R4S6 2004
    381'.456151'0973—dc22
                                                        2004013032

To Mary, always and all ways

CONTENTS

Foreword   ix
William L. Scharringhausen

Preface   xv

Acknowledgments   xvii

A Partial Chronology of Rexall   xx

PART I: THE LIGGETT LEGACY

Chapter 1. The Genius of Louis Liggett:
How It All Began   3

Chapter 2. "Dear Pardner"   17

Chapter 3. The Sense of Family and Its Effects:
Rexall Retirees Speak   27

PART II: MARKETING REXALL

Chapter 4. The Genius of Rexall Product   51

Chapter 5. The Genius of Rexall Price   67

Chapter 6. The Genius of Rexall Place   81

Chapter 7. The Genius of Rexall Promotion   113

PART III: THE DART ERA

Chapter 8. Justin Dart: A New Era of Genius   137

Chapter 9. The End of the Rexall Era   149

Chapter 10. Conclusion   155

Afterword   163

Appendix. A Profile of Hazard Rexall Drugs   165

Notes   171

Index   173

Foreword

"Why me?" seems to be a legitimate question in response to many of life's experiences—good, bad, and indifferent. Therefore, when Mickey Smith asked me to write the foreword to his book, "Why me?" was what I asked myself. Needless to say, I am flattered, honored, and humbled to be able to introduce you to *The Rexall Story: A History of Genius and Neglect*. A little personal background: I am proud to be a third-generation pharmacist. In Park Ridge, Illinois, in 1924, George L. Scharringhausen Sr., my grandfather, opened his own independent community pharmacy. (Was that not every pharmacist's dream?) His son, George L. Scharringhausen Jr., joined "Gramps" upon graduation from the University of Illinois College of Pharmacy in 1928. Mom and Dad's firstborn, my sister Helen, was also a pharmacist in the family business, after graduating from the University of Wisconsin School of Pharmacy in 1953. She continues to practice in Houston, Texas.

After graduating from the University of Wisconsin in 1956, I came on board. Scharringhausen Pharmacy obtained a Rexall franchise in the late 1920s (the old "blue" franchise), which offered the exclusive opportunity to buy and sell Rexall products in Park Ridge. Many after-school and weekend hours were spent dusting bottles and shelves, unpacking and putting away Rexall merchandise, and performing other necessary tasks, long before I was permitted to use the cash register. Was that not the goal of every youngster raised in a pharmacy family—to be able to "ring up a sale"?

Many pharmacy lessons and ethical business practices—as well as life lessons—were learned at the knees of my grandfather and father. Obviously, pharmacy and Rexall were in my blood from an early age. So I guess the "Why me?" is answered by Mickey's desire for someone with a strong Rexall background to introduce his book. I am also approaching my responsibility to the success of this book from the standpoint of a pharmacy family that was and is strongly involved in organizations that strive to make every pharmacy and pharmacist better—local, state, and national pharmacy associations. Dad was president of the Illinois Pharmacists Association and I was president of the National Asociation of Retail Druggists (NARD) (now the National Community Pharmacists Association [NCPA]), the national association representing the interests of independent community pharmacies. My commitment to their goals continues. Many other former Rexallites are equally, or better, qualified to write this foreword. Read on . . .

"Good Health to All from Rexall"

My Rexall experiences and recollections are many and varied. I recount many of them to pique your own interest and memories, whether you were a Rexallite or not. My comments are in no particular order, but it is appropriate to begin this trip through memory lane with mention of Rexall pharmaceuticals, the responsibility for many years of Joe Hailer. There was never a recall of a product from his department while he was in charge. Certainly, Rexall was a pioneer in the generic drug industry. Scharringhausen Pharmacy purchased Taladonna (phenobarbital and belladonna) tablets in drums of 5,000. Yes, our Park Ridge physicians prescribed a lot of Taladonna! It was economically, ethically, and professionally feasible for us to use Rexall products as extensively as possible.

Dad served on the Rexall Advisory Board in the late 1940s. Our family's first television set was purchased by Dad—I am sure as a bribe for my sister and me to behave while my grandmother took care of us on Mom and Dad's first trip to California for an advisory board meeting. Dad and other members of the board told it like it was, whether Rexall executives wanted to hear it or not. From the Rexallite's perspective, the advisory board served an important function. It was through his participation on the advisory board that Dad became well acquainted with many department heads. Names I recall that had much to do with Rexall's success were George Davis, Arch Carithers, and Howard Neill. Dad referred often to Louis K. Liggett and the company he started, United Wholesale Drug Company.

Liggett was a man of great foresight (genius?) who did much for the success of independent pharmacy. United Drug was a primary supplier to many Rexallites who were co-op members. I unpacked many large wooden United Drug/Rexall shipping crates filled with excelsior and Rexall merchandise. (We had some great incinerator fires with that excelsior!) Who can forget Cara-Nome Vanishing Cream; Mi31; Monacet Compound; Klenzo Mouthwash; US805 (rubbing alcohol); Reel-Roll Cotton; Quik-Bands; $50,000 Chocolate Syrup and Hot Fudge (served exclusively at our local country club and two fine restaurants because it was *the best*); Joan Manning chocolates; Kantleek (". . . on rubber is like sterling on silver"); and, of course, Bisma-Rex and Super Plenamins.

For many years, the only over-the-counter products that deserved a place on our wrapping/checkout counter were Rexall products. We were loyal to Rexall because Rexall was loyal to us. My Rexall memories would not be complete without mention of our super sales representatives, aka "Rexall reps," Al Leonard, Charlie Rhoten, Bernie Kay, and Bob Morelli, all of whom bled orange and blue blood in serving the Rexall stores in their territories. They truly were part of our family and were ever present in helping with display, promotion, sales associate training, and, dare I say, PMs (push monies). Their success translated into our success. Mention the Rexall One-Cent Sale and the conscience of an entire country is stirred. Twice a year, spring and fall, our little 1,500-square-foot pharmacy was transformed into the sale location of Park Ridge. With the help of sale tables and other displays made by my grandfather, Rexall's marketing expertise, and lots of hard work, we did one month's business in one week. Sale circulars, advance orders, signage on every retail store on Main Street, radio programs—such as *The Phil Harris/Alice Faye Show* and *Amos 'n' Andy*—and the opportunity for us to buy at sale prices did much to ensure our financial success.

Our promotion of One-Cent Sales and Rexall throughout the year made the names Scharringhausen and Rexall synonymous in our community. Some of my friends referred to me as "Billy Rexall," and some folks actually thought the symbol ℞ meant Rexall. For many years, our delivery vehicles were painted blue with an orange top and had the Rexall logo prominently displayed on both sides and the rear. At one of Rexall's many regional and state meetings, one of our employees (who incidentally earned enough PM to buy a fur coat) won a replica of a 1903 Oldsmobile complete with Rexall logo. For years that vehicle appeared in parades in our community.

All of these exciting times began to fade when we found that our exclusive franchise was no longer exclusive. The image and products for which we had established a high level of acceptance could not be purchased at other pharmacies where proprietors had no idea what made the image and products as good as they were. Eventually and unfortunately, "corporate Rexall," as with many other industries, became concerned with only bottom-line dollars, and not the Rexallites or the consumers it served. I believe that the demise of Rexall as we once knew it began when Rexall became a part of the Dart Industries pie. As the Rexall piece of that pie became smaller and smaller in the overall corporate structure, less and less attention (neglect?) was given to the issues that were important to Rexallites and the concept that got the whole business started. You need to read this book to get the entire story.

What about Pharmacy (capital P) and Independent Community Pharmacy today? The Rexall that we knew and loved would still be a successful franchise program. Opportunities to buy, sell, and promote an exclusive line of identifiable, quality drugstore merchandise with good profit margins and a trusted "We're in it for the long run" corporate attitude would ensure the viability of many an independent pharmacy. Along with the professional niches now available, which are signaling such new opportunities as diabetes, arthritis, hyperlipidemia, high blood pressure, men's health, counseling programs, and so on, the independent will survive and thrive. What is best for the patient and consumer must always be the bottom line. Because of the caliber of men and women who are pharmacists, the practice of Pharmacy (capital P) will continue to be America's Most Trusted Profession. It is important for us to be reminded of, and for future generations to know and to learn from, this part of the history that has made America great. The true Rexall reflected the values of us all, from the top-level corporate officer to the small-town American consumer.

Dad began writing a newsletter to our physicians when I was in pharmacy school. Eventually the mailing list included other pharmacy friends and associates in all phases of the profession and throughout the world. I continued to write it after his death in 1989 and until my retirement ten years later. He called the newsletter *Secundum Artem* (according to the art of the profession). *SA* was more than a name for a newsletter. It was the way Louis Liggett and

Joe Hailer and Scharringhausen Pharmacy and the thousands of other loyal Rexall employees and pharmacies and their employees conducted their business and lives. All of those relationships were built on trust. Rexallites trusted Rexall and our customers trusted us. Making a profit was an important and necessary consideration, but it was not the bottom line. Far more important was to have a good and ethical reputation in the industry and community. Sadly, corporate Rexall and, today, much of corporate America, lost sight of that.

Read, reflect, and enjoy *The Rexall Story: A History of Genius and Neglect*. I am proud to be a part of Mickey Smith's labor of love.

William L. Scharringhausen, RPh
Pharmacist, Rexallite, American

Preface

Good evening. This is your Rexall Family Druggist taking a little time from behind the prescription counter this Sunday evening to speak for all 10,000 of us, the 10,000 independent
druggists who have added the name Rexall to our own store
name. You can always tell us by the orange and blue sign on our
store windows. The sign means that we carry the 2,000 or more
drug products made by the Rexall Drug Company. They range
all the way from aspirins to penicillin, and they are as fine and
pure and dependable as science can make them. We independent druggists recommend them to our customers because we
know that you can always depend on a product that bears the
name Rexall.

This commercial message, delivered by the "Rexall Family Druggist" at the conclusion of *The Phil Harris/Alice Faye Show* radio
broadcast on February 6, 1949, illustrates two points important to this
account: First, Rexall knew how to advertise. One must hear the voice
of this kindly gentleman to fully appreciate the sincerity with which
the message was delivered. More about him and other Rexall promotions appears later in the book. Second, but most important and the
compelling reason for writing this, is mention of the 10,000 Rexall
druggists. Now there are none. Once they represented one-fifth of all
drugstores! *Were* they dinosaurs that disappeared without explanation? I do not promise a definitive answer. Indeed, I expect some dis-
agreement, but it is my hope that the story of the disappearance of a
part of Americana will be worth the reading.

Acknowledgments

This book originated as a consequence of the serendipitous confluence of hobbies and a shared profession. Frank Sternad of Fullerton, California, has long been collecting Rexall memorabilia. His classified ads in *The American Journal of the History of Pharmacy* first attracted my attention as a result of my own hobby, collecting recordings of "classic" radio. Critical to the first contact was my admiration for the way Rexall handled its sponsorship of *The Phil Harris/Alice Faye Show.*

Many phone calls, e-mails, and letters followed, and I owe a great debt to Frank for his many ideas, tips, and suggestions. That our respective visions of the nature and scope of a history of Rexall eventually meant a separation of efforts in no way diminishes my respect for his great efforts, knowledge, and assistance.

A number of Rexall retirees have provided vital insights, either by phone or letter, as well as copies of company documents and communications. I have not identified them by name in association with comments and quotations in the book but do so here. The list includes all who helped. It is impossible to list especially helpful contributions without the risk of offending someone, so I acknowledge each individually in alphabetical order: William Blaine, Don Boughn, Norma Bowles, Forrest Bush, W. E. Cochran, Landis Eby, Jeanne Frett, R. H. Garrison, Ralph Garner, Richard Green, Laverne B. Hawkinson, William Heyler, Jack Hopkins, Verl Kersey, Peg Lambert, Don Latta, Juan Ledo, John Little, Jim Neilson, Rex Oehm, W. T. Ozmint, Ernie Parker, Ruth Pohlman, Louise Saulvester, Bill Scharringhausen, Dick Seymour, Ted Trump, Howard VanderLinden, and Tom Zangriles.

Two graduate students, Don Dickerson and David Scheffler, were a great help in research, as were the historians at the American Institute of the History of Pharmacy and Jill Nissen at the library of the St. Louis College of Pharmacy.

John Kallir helped with referrals and by publicizing this effort in the *Healthcare Marketing and Communications Council Newsletter.*

Mississippi pharmacists Aston Holley, Clint Johnson, and Luck Wing contributed memories, and, of course, I am in debt to Joe and Elizabeth Duncan for permission to share the story of Hazard Rexall Drugs.

Linda Rike helped in many ways, especially early in the project, and Colleen McPherson did a super job in preparing the manuscript.

Finally, my wife Mary has been a constant source of encouragement, constructive criticism, new ideas and perspectives, and, as with my previous books, *patience.*

Errors, omissions, and other flaws can and should be assigned to only me.

ABOUT THE AUTHOR

Mickey C. Smith, PhD, is Professor Emeritus in the School of Pharmacy at the University of Mississippi. He is a highly acclaimed researcher/writer with an international reputation in the field of pharmaceutical marketing. Dr. Smith is the principal author and editor of *Pharmaceutical Marketing: Principles, Environment and Practices,* the only textbook of its kind. He has published more than 400 articles in more than 100 different research and professional journals, is Co-Editor in Chief of Pharmaceutical Products Press, an imprint of The Haworth Press, Inc., and is Founding Editor of the *Journal of Pharmaceutical Marketing and Management.* Dr. Smith was named Mississippi's Professor of the Year for 1993, an honor conferred annually on one college instructor per state by the Council for Advancement and Support of Education (CASE) in Washington. Other various awards include the Research Achievement Award from the Academy of Pharmaceutical Sciences, the Rho Chi national lecture award, the first-ever Lyman Award, the first-ever Distinguished Educator Award from the American Association of Colleges of Pharmacy, and, from the University of Mississippi, the Burlington-Northern Award. His research interests range from health planning and health economics to the sociological aspects of pharmacy.

A PARTIAL CHRONOLOGY OF REXALL

Company Names and Other Significant Dates
Through Rexall History

	1902-1911	United Drug Company is incorporated in New Jersey in 1902.
United Drug Company is incorporated in Massachusetts in 1911.	**1911-1916**	
	1916-1928	United Drug Company is incorporated in Massachusetts in 1916.
United Drug Company is incorporated in Delaware in 1928.	**1928**	
	1941	Louis Liggett retires from active service and is succeeded by Joseph Galvin. Justin Dart is hired.
Justin Dart is elected president of United Drug.	**1943**	
	1945	Name is changed to United-Rexall Drug Company. Headquarters move to Los Angeles is completed and reorganization begins.
Death of Louis Liggett.	**1946**	
	1947	Name is changed to Rexall Drug Company.
John Bowles becomes Rexall President.	**1955**	
	1958	Rexall buys Tupperware.

Name is changed to Rexall Drug and Chemical Company.	1959	
	1969	Name is changed to Dart Industries, Inc.
		Failed attempt is made to sell Rexall to Commonwealth.
Rexall Drug Company incorporated in Delaware in 1969 (operated the Rexall business as a wholly owned subsidiary of Dart Industries, Inc.).	1970-1976	
	1977	Rexall is sold to Ross-Hall.
Rexall Drug Company incorporated in Delaware in 1976 (a closely-held, private corporation—Ross-Hall).	1977-1981	
	1980	Dart and Kraft merge. All Rexall franchises are canceled by Weber.
Death of Justin Dart.	1984	
	1986	Rexall is acquired by Sundown.

PART I:
THE LIGGETT LEGACY

Chapter 1

The Genius of Louis Liggett:
How It All Began

Louis Kohl Liggett was:
  a. A business genius.
  b. An opportunist.
  c. Someone with an idea whose time had come and who recognized it.
  d. Someone who invented a time for an idea to come.
  e. A humanitarian.
  f. Someone who genuinely believed that he could "do well by doing good."
  g. A charismatic speaker.

If you answered, "All of the above," history would seem to support you.[1]

Early on in work on this book, it seemed obvious that Liggett should be described as someone out of the pages of Horatio Alger. I was given pause by an article in *The Wall Street Journal* (August 27, 2003, p. 81) which suggested that Alger's books, in contrast to the widely held stereotype of his heroes, actually portrayed men (always men) who, according to the article, "rarely became wealthy by Gilded Age standards, and most didn't even aspire to great fortunes. They wanted to join the middle class that was slowly developing in America, and become comfortable, secure and upwardly mobile."

Well, Liggett did, in fact, fit the stereotype of "people who have risen from poverty to success, using bootstraps, hard work, and fair play." He transformed the retail drug business for a half century, and some believe that transformation would continue today, but for a series of decisions that will be described in due course.

Liggett got his start in the drug business selling a patent medicine tonic named Vinol. He was twenty-five years old at the turn of the twentieth century when he demonstrated to his general manager that he could not only sell the product (ten gross during his first week on the job) but also had a scheme to do even better.

After learning that some of his Vinol agents were selling the product at cut-rate prices, he concluded that exclusivity, not competition, was the answer to increased sales. Only one outlet in any city should be allowed to sell Vinol. No *need* to cut the prices. The Rexall franchise was already germinating, although "Rexall" was yet to be born and named. In the meantime, Liggett was honing his natural personal and merchandising skills on behalf of Vinol.

Liggett traveled the entire country. It is clear that his customers liked and trusted him. He was not just a salesman, but rather a partner in the Vinol business. He provided valuable suggestions to his customers on how to sell Vinol. These suggestions, which worked, were appreciated.

During this time, events and practices foreshadowing the Rexall era were taking place. Liggett formed a Vinol Club (later there would be the International Rexall Clubs). He published the *Vinol Voice,* presaging the *Rexall Ad-Vantages*. Most important, however, he diagnosed a need—or an *opportunity* among retail druggists. According to one account, he began his revolution at a Vinol Club meeting in Buffalo in 1901 where he organized the Drug Merchants of America. It had no connection with Vinol. The premise was so simple that it seems obvious today.

Typical of Liggett throughout his remarkable career, he began by seeing someone else's problem, in this case the druggist who was paying a substantial part of potential profit to jobbers and wholesalers. Liggett's plan? To sell to one druggist in each town at factory prices. The factory, which did not exist, would sell its merchandise under a private label (later to be called "own goods").

So far, Liggett had just an idea—no factory, no merchandise, and no capital. At this time, his personal integrity and believability became his capital. His first contact was James DeMoville in Nashville, who, in what must have been a very persuasive buggy ride to the Hermitage, was moved to great enthusiasm. He was to become the first of the original forty stockholders. The second was T. P. Taylor in Louisville, Kentucky. Again, Liggett used personal persuasion away from the drugstore.

So here was the challenge: two enthusiastic supporters and a strong belief in a concept, but no money! Again, the Liggett personality came to his (and Pharmacy's) rescue. With DeMoville's help he organized a meeting of the forty original stockholders of what was to become the United Drug Company. These forty men, "the foremost druggists in the country," (p. 1)[2] were chosen and contacted by seven of Liggett's druggist friends. Incredibly, given the times, each agreed to invest $4,000 in a company that was still just an idea.

Liggett crafted his idea into a policy that included the following principles:

1. The company should manufacture controlled-brand goods only for its stockholder agents.
2. There would be no more than one controlling member in any one city or town in the United States.
3. The company would manufacture its own products under its own trade names.
4. These products would be sold to the agent/stockholder at a price sufficient to net the company a reasonable profit.
5. Control of the products would remain in the hands of the druggists themselves.

The following list of those original forty stockholders illustrates the broad commercial and private representation at the start of this venture.

Wolff-Wilson Drug Co.	St. Louis, Missouri
Stephen Hester	Chicago, Illinois
Adolph Speigel	Milwaukee, Wisconsin
W. G. Marshall	Cleveland, Ohio
A. W. M. Moffitt	Troy, New York
Charles A. Rapelye	Hartford, Connecticut
Byron M. Hyde	Rochester, New York
E. L. Scholtz	Denver, Colorado
James L. DeMoville	Nashville, Tennessee
Wm. B. Riker & Son Co.	New York, New York
W. C. Bolton	Brooklyn, New York

William Sautter	Albany, New York
J. C. Brady	Fall River, Massachusetts
Voegeli Bros. Drug Co.	Minneapolis, Minnesota
May Drug Co.	Pittsburgh, Pennsylvania
E. R. Petty	Newark, New Jersey
Columbus Pharmacal Co.	Columbus, Ohio
Jennie Hamilton Pharmacy	Bridgeport, Connecticut
C. E. Ball Drug Co.	Holyoke, Massachusetts
Gray and Worcester	Detroit, Michigan
L. M. Reed and Son	Toledo, Ohio
T. P. Taylor and Son	Louisville, Kentucky
George C. Lyon	Providence, Rhode Island
Henry C. Hall	Waltham, Massachusetts
Peck Bros.	Grand Rapids, Michigan
C. H. and H. A. Lawton	New Bedford, Massachusetts
Hayes and Pierson Co.	Fitchburg, Massachusetts
W. H. Curier and Co.	Pittsfield, Massachusetts
Faxon, Williams & Faxon	Buffalo, New York
Jaynes Drug Co.	Buffalo, New York
H. D. Dwight & Co.	Syracuse, New York
John W. Miller	Dayton, Ohio
Averbeck Drug Co.	Youngstown, Ohio
Louis K. Liggett	Boston, Massachusetts
James T. Weatherald	Boston, Massachusetts
H. J. Huder	Indianapolis, Indiana
W. M. Federmann	Kansas City, Missouri
Sherman & McConnell	Omaha, Nebraska
Hall and Lyon Co.	Worcester, Massachusetts
Druehl and Franken	Salt Lake City, Utah

The first president of the company was E. D. Cahoon of the Wm. B. Riker & Son Company of New York (the names of Cahoon and Riker will figure again in this history), DeMoville was second vice president, J. T. Weatherald was treasurer, and Liggett was secretary and general manager.

The original group chose the name "Saxona" for their products-to-be, but W. T. Wilson, Liggett's "office boy," suggested an alternative: Rexall—"king" of all. *Brilliant!* Of course, any pharmacist also knows that Rx stands for prescription. Thus, the name suggested two meanings, both of them very marketable.

Liggett spent most of that original $160,000 on promotional ventures to create public curiosity about the name *Rexall*. He also leased a vacant building in Boston in which to manufacture Rexall products, from which in early 1903 the first shipment departed.

A bit of the spirit of P. T. Barnum now appeared. By late 1903 there were 172 stockholders who met for their first convention. Liggett organized his smartly attired employees in the first shop scheduled to be seen by the visiting stockholders. As the visitors filed out, the employees quickly moved on to the next shop on the factory tour. Apparently, no one noticed that the same employees reappeared throughout the different factory visits.

In a report to his agents in 1904, Liggett chronicled the progress in the previous year. The number of employees had increased from 0 to 241, and sales had risen from $0 to $61,777—quite an impressive beginning. Also during this year, Liggett and the company took a paradoxical step. They opened a drugstore of their own, which was, of course, in contrast to the original franchise-only policy. The move foreshadowed what was to be a major venture into retail ownership, one that would create what was, at one time, the largest retail drug chain in the country.

Liggett was a great communicator and extremely persuasive. He firmly believed in his company and also in expansion. Candy was part of his product line from the very beginning. Then in 1905 he formed the National Cigar Stands company. Though not a part of United Drug, it allowed United agents to purchase tobacco products at reduced prices. Liggett was accused by United Cigar Stores of trying to monopolize the tobacco business. Their efforts to stop this expansion failed, but Liggett would be involved in many legal and business battles throughout his career.

One such battle involved the acquisition of a chain of drugstores, interesting because the chains were considered to be the most serious threat to the survival of the independent pharmacists who constituted the franchise/stockholder clientele of United Drug. Then the man described as having "done more for the retail drug stores than has any other living man"[3] seemed bent on doing even more.

By 1916 a new L. K. Liggett Company had been formed and had control of 152 retail stores, but it had not been easy. The Riker drug chain had acquired the Hegeman chain, causing anxiety among independents in the area served by Riker, and earlier, in 1910, J. B. Cobb, representing Riker, demanded to know the reason for the formation of the Liggett Company and, as a stockholder in United Drug, tried in vain to convince the United board against Liggett. Liggett responded with a proposal to merge Riker and United Drug, but that was rejected. The details of the legal wrangling are relevant but not essential to this story. What *is* essential is the knowledge that (this time with Cobb's agreement), by 1916, the Liggett organization owned those 152 stores and had franchise agreements with nearly 6,000 other stores. And Liggett wasn't finished.

In 1912 Liggett had traveled to England, where he organized 126 stockholders along the lines of the company in the United States. Typical of the man, he interviewed each of those men personally. He would return to England with even more ambitious plans.

Throughout the early decade, expansion and acquisition continued. The first Liggett-built store, at Broadway and Thirty-Fourth Street in Manhattan, was opened. The Guth Chocolate Company was acquired, as was United Cigar Stores which until then had been a loose relationship from which the company had not profited.

Liggett also continued his efforts to assist his franchisees in achieving success. He established salesmanship courses for their staff and *Rexall Magazine,* which was filled with ads, of course, but also puzzles and other entertainment. By 1919 the magazine had achieved a circulation of 1.3 million! He supported prohibition even though his stores did $180,000 annually in the liquor business, figuring that the loss in business would be offset by goodwill. Attempting to garner further goodwill in various circles, Liggett set up a special block of stock for franchise salespeople; he suggested free prescriptions for the "worthy poor"; and he removed the four Rexall products containing narcotics after the Harrison Narcotic Act took effect in 1915.

The Seamless Rubber Company and Hanson-Jacks (perfumes) were acquired in 1917, when the United States entered World War I. Liggett's response? He made an offer to the Secretary of War offering the services of Rexallites as recruiting agents for the military. He also purchased a 100-foot cruiser that he rented to the U.S. Navy as a subchaser for $1.00 a year. In addition, he enlisted his Rexallites in a fight against the growing spread of venereal disease. Each signed a pledge "not to prescribe or recommend any remedy for venereal disease and not to purchase any such remedy" (Rexall ms., p. 26).

By 1920 the company had so impressed the business community that Richardson, Hill and Company, a New York stockbroker, had this to say in a public letter:

UNITED DRUG COMPANY

Industrial or Public Utility
In all seriousness it may be asked whether the business of the United Drug Company, with the unique relation which its chain of stores bears to the needs of the people, is not to be classed as a quasi-public institution. It is to the drug store that people in all walks of life instinctively turn for assistance in accidents, for relief in illness, for help in emergencies, at all hours of the day and night, and while this has been true from the days of the mortar and pestle apothecary shop, it is so in an entirely new sense today, owing to the rapid evolution of the Liggett system of production and distribution.

For this organization apparently has the inclination and the ability to originate, manufacture and distribute a variety of articles contributing to the physical well-being of both sexes and every age, limited only by the character of the demand, which must be national to get recognition. Thus it is that the man in the street today demands a Liggett store conveniently near his location, wherever he may happen to be, as a first-aid station, not only to administer to his needs in illness, but to his comfort when in health as well. Liggett stores are in their way as much an urban utility as are libraries and trolley lines.

Also in 1920 came the acquisition of England's Boot's Drug Company. The war had been financially damaging for both Liggett and Boot's, but worse for the latter. A dying Sir Jesse Boot was ready to sell, and Liggett was ready to buy. He acquired 627 of "Boot's Cash Chemists," a manufacturing facility in Nottingham that he needed, and important connections in other countries still nominally part of the British "Empire." Back in 1912, after his visit to England, Liggett said, "I found that if any American Company expects to succeed in England and develop its business they had better start in playing the piccolo rather than a brass band" (*The Pharmaceutical Era,* June 1912). Liggett had just bought a brass band.

United opened its own manufacturing plant in St. Louis in 1920, but 1921 proved to be a major trial. The stock market was in bad shape, but United Drug stock was in worse condition, showing a price drop from a high of $106 to $46 per share. True to form, Liggett tried desperately to protect his own and his stockholders' interests. An urgent appeal was sent to Rexallites not to sell, and Liggett spent his entire fortune buying stock that he used as collateral for loans to buy more. Here was a man who put his money where his mouth was. Unfortunately, his money was gone; he was financially ruined. At this point we can truly see the influence of his personal integrity and encouragement on his colleagues in the company.

The response to the Liggett financial disaster is almost certainly unparalleled in major corporate history. Upon learning of his plight, the International Rexall Clubs, under the leadership of then President Harry Dockum, did two things:

1. They started a big drive to sell more Rexall products, and the results were astounding. A 40 percent club was organized to include all agents who gave United Drug 40 percent of all their purchases.
2. Even more remarkable, a Rexall Loyalty Trust Fund was formed to raise $3 million to pull Liggett out of debt. They did it. The crisis that might have spelled the end of Rexall was over, and the progress continued.

In 1925 Rexall entered into a contract with Owl Drug Stores of Southern California. Owl agreed to give United a percentage of its sales in return for Rexall advertising. The agreement didn't last, however, as competition forced Owl to lower the percentage of business accorded to United. The contract was canceled, and Rexall agencies replaced Owl Drug Stores in Southern California. In 1930, however, United did purchase the 108-store chain.

The year 1928 brought another major merger, this time between United and Sterling Products. Sterling was big. They had patents on Bayer Aspirin, Danderine, and others. The two companies had almost equal earnings, but United had the greater sales volume.

Liggett had eyes on Bristol-Myers and hoped that the merger with Sterling would provide the muscle. They added Phillips' Milk of Magnesia and, in 1926, Ipana Tooth Paste and Sal Hepatica, manufactured by Bristol-Myers. (Years later a radio theme would be "Ipana for the smile of beauty. Sal Hepatica for the smile of health.") The list of other acquisitions was remarkable. Among them were Life Savers, 3-in-1 Oil, Fletcher's Castoria, and Mum.

Then came 1929 and the crash of the stock market. While United remained relatively solid, the L.K. Liggett Company was slipping inevitably into bankruptcy, which occurred in 1933. Meanwhile, in 1932, Liggett had offered six months credit at 3 percent to help bail out his beloved franchisers, and many were, indeed, saved.

The year 1933 also saw the dissolution of the Sterling agreement. Rexall agents were not happy with Sterling, and Sterling apparently resented the close "family" ties between the agents and United. In an effort to raise capital, Liggett began to look to Boot's in England.

After negotiations frustrated by English Prime Minister Neville Chamberlain's insistence that the deal could not go through, a deal was finally approved, and through a series of complicated maneuvers, Liggett was allowed to sell Boot's and take his money home. His "money" was $32-plus million, compared with his original purchase price of $10 million—not bad, as it was now possible to buy back the Liggett drug chain. Nevertheless, for the first time in its history, United operated at a loss.

In 1935 United established a new Department of Research and Technology with the stated purpose of doing extensive research in the field of pharmacy. Then in 1936 one of the most flamboyant promotions in the history of the company was conducted: the Rexall Train, described as "a convention in itself." By now there were nearly 7,600 Rexall druggists, and a convention was out of the question, so the decision was made to bring the convention to them.

The train covered nearly 30,000 miles and visited 150 cities, stopping for one day each for business meetings. Leased from the Pullman Company, the train embodied the Rexall organization. Twelve air-conditioned (!) streamlined cars, each with its own particular purpose, were involved. One was a modern drugstore with a soda fountain. Another contained a full-scale model of Rexall's plants and brands. Yet another showed a model of the research facilities. Living quarters for Liggett were also included. A bright blue exterior and the words "The Rexall Train" appeared on the train (more to follow in Chapter 7 on promotion).

All of Rexall's customers, the agents, and the general public had a look. The mornings featured business sessions with the stockholders, followed by public tours. The evenings offered dining and dancing for the stockholders and their families. Nothing like this had been seen before, or since.

Progress continued apace during the 1930s, and in 1939 the biggest One-Cent Sale in the history of the company was celebrated (much more on the One-Cent Sale in Chapter 5 on pricing). Another big event was the Rexallite Convention held at the San Francisco World's Fair. Reports say that it resembled a political convention. After viewing an exhibit of United Drug merchandise, the registrants gathered in the convention hall amid much pandemonium. With trumpets and white horses, a parade was executed in tribute to Louis Liggett, followed by a several-minute ovation before Mr. Liggett could speak.

In 1941 Liggett retired from active service as president of United Drug and was succeeded by Joseph Galvin, in whom Liggett expressed great confidence in his final "Dear Pardner" letter (see Chapter 2). By now, United Drug owned nearly 600 drugstores and boasted nearly 8,000 Rexall franchisees, 16,000 employees, and 5,000 products. This was also the year Justin Dart was hired. (Dart deserves, and will receive, individual attention in later chapters).

Then came Pearl Harbor and World War II—The Big One. Two United subsidiaries, the Absorbent Cotton Company (bandages) and the Seamless Rubber Company (rubber products), earned the Army-Navy "E" Award for excellence in promoting the war effort. Another subsidiary, a candy plant, produced tons of K rations. Liggett must certainly have been very proud.

In 1945 Liggett took a final farewell, becoming honorary chairman of the board after forty-three years of service to the company and inspiration to his "Pardners" and stockholders. Table 1.1 presents the (incomplete) record of his accomplishments. These statistics only begin to capture the incredible scope of Liggett's accomplishments, many of them achieved by dint of enthusiasm, persuasiveness, and absolute belief in his mission and the people around him.

TABLE 1.1. Growth of United/Rexall Retail Business

Year	Agencies	Liggett	Owl	Sontag	Liggett Canada	Total Company-Owned Stores
1903	279					
1904	767					
1905	833					
1906	1,081					
1907	1,360					
1908	1,762					
1909	2,218					
1910	2,755					
1911	3,628					
1912	4,534					
1913	5,056					
1914	5,570					
1915	5,877					
1916	5,981					
1917	6,259					
1918	6,344					
1919	6,402					
1920	6,650					
1921	6,981					
1922	7,272					
1923	7,360					
1924	7,356					
1925	7,365					
1926	7,302					
1927	7,229					
1928	7,276					
1929	7,347					

TABLE 1.1 *(continued)*

1930	7,324					
1931	7,234					
1932	7,457					
1933	7,584					
1934	7,637	449	108		43	600
1935	7,592	449	121		45	615
1936	7,587	448	122		45	615
1937	7,584	449	129		49	627
1938	7,604	433	128		50	611
1939	7,642	425	129		50	604
1940	7,625	415	132		50	597
1941	7,749	402	133		49	584
1942	7,904	392	134		47	573
1943	7,920	381	142		45	568
1944	7,954	364	132	50	44	590
1945	8,141	342	122	48	48	558
1946	8,300	307	164	Combined with Owl	48	594

Source: Rexall ms.
Note: Numbers and dates are approximate.

In a letter to stockholders in 1920, Liggett finished with the following:

> Never in the Company's history has it been as strong as it is today. Its finances, equipment, and organization have been improved wherever possible and its trademarks have risen in public esteem.
>
> The intangible values being accumulated, including long leaseholds for stores in prominent locations, are not shown in profits, but in my opinion they have grown to be worth more than all the physical property put together, and I ask you to witness the future to confirm this judgment.

This was vintage Liggett, and surely history *did* confirm his judgment. Certainly no CEO of any major corporation has made such an effort to maintain personal contact with his customers and stockholders as did Liggett. His eloquence deserves special attention, which will be supplied in Chapter 2.

Liggett received many honors, among them an honorary Doctor of Pharmacy degree from the Rhode Island College of Pharmacy. He died in 1946 after more than four decades as the Father of Rexall.

Chapter 2

"Dear Pardner"

According to Merwin (*RFA,* p. 64), Liggett wrote 268 Dear Pardner letters between the time he started in 1903 and 1923. The total number is not documented, but his last was the announcement that his health would not permit him to continue in an active role with the company he had built and nurtured.

So what were the Dear Pardner letters? They were (and are) without precedent in "big business." An example from his letter of April 8, 1914: "It's been a long time since we had a heart-to-heart talk. Maybe I have neglected my duty as President of your company in not writing to you more frequently." Liggett told his readers ("Pardners") that he had just heard from one of his stockholders: "Mr. Liggett, the loyal stockholders of the United Drug Company want to hear from you." This personal relationship was apparently not shared by all, and Liggett, who gave every evidence of his personal concern for his Pardners, could be tough as well.

In the same letter, Liggett expressed astonishment at the fact that about 500 shareholders were not, based on their orders, loyal to the company. "In other words, they were being carried along by the 5,000 stockholders who are supporting the organization." Liggett made a (not too) veiled threat to "take action on the whole list of stockholders who have not during the past twelve months properly supported this organization." He was totally committed and expected the same from his Pardners.

His first letter (date undocumented) is worth repeating verbatim. (*RFA,* pp. 67-69):

DEAR PARDNER:

Having resigned some time ago the editorship of *Vinol Voice,* I now find myself burdened with an innate feeling to again come in close touch with you, and, therefore, from now on I shall burden you with a semi-monthly letter.

The literature embodied in these letters will pertain most to REXALL, but I shall occasionally remember, if possible, that you handle other products, and if I can borrow or steal any ideas in my travels that I think will assist you in advancing your business outside of REXALL, I will add it in without charge. I'll not do this because I want to help you push other products, but I know that any plans which may assist your general business will make you feel more interested in REXALL, especially if they come through this office. Now that I have given you fair warning of what is to come every fortnight, I'll dig down to letter number one.

We, the stockholders of the U. D. Co., are pardners (therein you will find my excuse for addressing you as above) and naturally you will expect an occasional report from the General Manager.

I am told that our company has stirred up considerable conversation throughout the country, and some of the remarks that have been overheard have made me realize that some jealous people can say mean things, but to date, I must confess that I am surprised that they haven't been meaner. On the other hand the nice things we hear about our advertising and style of packages make me feel that there is more sunshine than clouds in the U. D. Co.'s sky.

Touching on the advertising questions, I want to say a few words about our Rexall work. Some of you have wondered how we were going to make a 25c [c = cent] Dyspepsia Cure pay for all the big space we are using. Didn't you realize that your Executive Committee had carefully considered this subject? Did you not see that we were first aiming to introduce the word "REXALL," second to sell Dyspepsia Cure, and won't you now agree with us in thinking that your Executive Committee was right, that the daily spelling of the word REXALL* cost money, but didn't it catch in your town? And isn't it today a word that is as well known to the drug buyers as almost any medicine you have on your shelf? And think of it, we've only been at the game ten weeks, yet Rexall is established in the minds of the people and it has left a pleasing impression too with the clever "kids" and Captain Rexall, to say nothing of the great prominence given your store—that is one point you must not overlook, no matter how much or how little Dyspepsia Cure you have sold.

---

* Liggett had run a series of ads, the first beginning with a very large "R," the second with an "E," and so on until he had built curiosity, which was satisfied when REXALL was revealed.

This brings another point to my mind. Are you taking advantage of this great Rexall campaign by pushing the "trailers"? You must admit they are a clever line of articles—and such a low price on them. It makes me feel sick sometimes to see the company's profit compared alongside of yours on these articles, and it's easy for you to sell them—only a window display and a little push from behind the counter. You are taking advantage of the advertising when you do this.

But getting back to Rexall Dyspepsia Cure. This article is going to be a big winner, and in the end is going to pay the bills for introducing the word Rexall.

We're getting down to solid dyspepsia talk in the newspapers now, and with a goodly list of testimonials accumulating every day we will soon fill the space with "stuff" that will "cut ice."

We're going on the bill boards in July with the greatest poster out; twelve and one sheets galore, and there won't be a man, woman, or child in your town July 4th but what will have an intimate acquaintance with Captain Rexall and her kids. Here again is your opportunity to push the trailers. These posters will sell a world of them if you'll only help.

Now I know you're aching for some news of the inside working of the laboratory. We're in good running order now. Just five months ago we had a bare building, five floors with over six thousand feet to a floor. We wondered how we were going to fill it; and now we're wondering what we are going to do for more manufacturing room next fall.

So as to show you that we've not been asleep I will give you some figures. On February last we had a dozen employees, on March 1st we had sixty, and today we are pushing to the one hundred and fifty mark. From March 15th to April 15th we turned out 200,000 packages of Dyspepsia Cure, making the tablets, boxes, labels, booklets and everything pertaining to the package in our own plant.

We have kept our Printing Dep't with its four big presses and six printers a full month behind in their work. We have increased our stockholders from 40 to 251 (more agents than there were for Vinol at the end of their third year). We have kept our electrotype foundry running steadily until long after hours, to say nothing of our Advertising Manager; we've made an owl of him, and we haven't made any costly mistakes as far as we can see today.

We have designed, and made entirely in our plant, fifty complete packages of patent medicine—that was no small task, almost one a day, and of the whole lot we had trouble with one formula only. Doesn't that speak well for our department heads and their ability to get good work out of their employees?

Some of you will say; "Well, you've not filled our orders yet." That's true—we've had lots to contend with. 1st: The tin box proposition; that's all right now. 2nd: Glassware for tooth powder; that's all right now. 3rd: A new concern with over 200 fellows all wanting their goods at one time naturally brings a delay on something. Forgive us if we've disappointed you, but from now on blame us, and don't hesitate if orders are not out on time.

I don't want you to think that we are looking for praise (although in entertaining over fifty visiting stockholders we aren't less happy for their praises, and one can't help but feel that we've given results so far when such men as Mr. Hexter, Mr. Spiegel, Mr. Jaynes, Mr. Bolton and a dozen other big fellows ask us how we did it). It's not that reason I have in mind in writing you all this; it's to impress upon you that you have a big—yes—a great big plant down here that can turn out tons of medicine, and that it's now "up to you" to keep it going so that we can all get a profit. It's the volume of business that will count now. You must not lay back on the oars and say, "You fellows have got our money, now see what you can do." We've done it—and we're going to do more, but what we want is your push on the trailers.

Tom Taylor of Louisville was here yesterday. He says the plant is just the thing for his business. So impressed was he with the new list of trailers that he gave us an order of 100 to 1,000 of every article on the list.

Mr. Hexter of Chicago who has been here says he'll give us $1,000 a month from now on for trailers. Think of it; if these men, with the big competition they have, find it an advantage to plug the Rexall trailers, isn't it money in your pocket to do the same?

Look at our prices again, please. There is Toothache Gum, about $2.00 per hundred packages. There are 250 of you stockholders. Why not each take 100, that's $500 to us. Now average that whole list up and see what a money making proposition we have as a combination, and when that list goes to 100 articles, which it will by October 1st, we will keep 200 families living off the U. D. Co.'s payroll.

I know you take pride in this plant, and when you come to the Stockholders' Meeting (which you must not fail to do) September 29th and 30th, I feel certain that you will go back knowing that your investment was not a mistake.

There are a dozen more things I want to write about, but you're tired, so am I, and therefore I will close with my kind regards and best hopes for another order on trailers soon.

Yours very sincerely,
LOUIS K. LIGGETT

P.S. Don't know what my next letter will be on, but I've a few remarks to make on window display and candy. Because I've talked "trailers," don't forget Dyspepsia Cure. July 1st window displays will back up the posters.

Q.S. The Executive Committee will soon formally announce the Stockholders' Meeting. I didn't intend to give away the secret, but it's out now. The date is September 29th and 30th, and it's for both Common and Preferred, and there'll be some "doings" besides business.

L. K. L.

So that's how it began: this personal communication between a man who was to become a major U.S. industrialist and the people who depended on his leadership and on whom he depended for business success. Liggett was always teaching, always explaining. Perhaps he was paternalistic, but he never seemed to talk down to his audience, even though, truthfully, he knew more than most of them did about the business.

When United was sued by a small company with a history of using the word *Rex,* it was obviously not a matter of great concern to Liggett, who told his stockholders ("Dear Pardner," February 11, 1916), "This suit is one of the penalties of growing and progressing. There are people in this world who are looking for easy money, and strive as you may, sometimes they will catch you napping." The lawsuit would probably be considered a "nuisance suit" by today's standards, but given the future importance of the Rexall trademark (which even Liggett could not possibly have foreseen), the possible ramifications were serious. His response was more or less, "Don't worry. Be happy. I'll take care of this." And he did.

In January 1914 Liggett wrote to his Pardners about their efforts to influence a repeal of the war tax on perfumes, toiletries, and cosmetics. By his account, some 15,000 Rexallites had written to Congress on the matter. He acknowledged the work of the (then) National Association of Retail Druggists but also added a note of restraint:

> To those of you who have suggested that we use our influence toward other legislation, let me say that it would be very poor policy for the United Drug Company to interest itself in any legislation that doesn't affect Rexallites as a whole. Any attempt to use our organization toward individual class or individual sec-

tion legislation would, in my opinion, destroy the value of the present influence.

This lifelong Republican did not omit some advice on the business. Noting the individual sale in the drugstore was but twenty-three cents, according to reports, he advised his Pardners to "take a grip on things. GO TO IT."

In a March 1915 letter addressed individually to one Pardner he asked why the addressee was not insured with the United Druggists Mutual Fire Insurance Company. Again, a very personal letter explained the savings accruing to Rexallites:

> It's easy enough for me to build this Insurance Company up to a big business by taking outside insurance. We are not doing this—we are operating this Insurance Company for the benefit of Rexall Stockholders. Our chances for conflagration are minimized because of the fact that we have only one stockholder in each community. This fact makes us a *very strong* Company. Furthermore, we know the people we are insuring; we are *ONE BIG FAMILY*—the larger we can make this family, the cheaper we can write your insurance.

In March 1917 Liggett (and everyone) saw war on the horizon. He canceled the conventions and explained that to his Pardners. In August of the same year he explained to them how, legally, to recommend the United Drug brand of aspirin, for which the patent had expired. Bayer had owned the patent, but trademark implications required explanation. The explanation was accompanied by an order form—a bottle of twenty-four for fifteen cents.

In 1918 he stepped up his war efforts, enlisting Rexallites to recruit men for the merchant marines. By March of that year, he had supplied everyone with recruiting materials. Although he had to give them a strong nudge in his letters of April 11 and May 28, ultimately, United's campaign was a major success. Also in 1918, he asked, in an impassioned letter, for his pharmacists to cooperate in a fight against venereal disease—another success and great public relations as well.

By January 1921 Liggett was giving his Pardners a lesson on the workings of distribution channels. Postwar times were tough, but Liggett had some answers:

It is true that supply and demand make business. We also can make demand by effort, when otherwise it would not come. The retailer is the neck of the bottle through which merchandise eventually flows. When he corks up, as he has been corked up for the past five or six months, everything backs up—factories stop—people are out of employment—but the retailer has got to take care of demand. His stocks determine production; as soon as he begins to buy, factories begin to run. If we step on the throttle and go after business from the retailer's standpoint, we will find 1921 to be one of the largest years in volume and in profits that we have ever had. What we want to do is to increase our stock turn-over by carrying a minimum of stocks, both retail and manufacturing.

In April of the same year, Liggett was selling United stock, encouraging the drugstore owners who were already shareholders to seek buyers of stock from among their clerks, customers, friends, and physicians. The premise was clever indeed! The more stockholders in town, the more potential business. As Liggett noted:

[T]he stockholders you now get among your friends should be the representative people in your communities—people who can do you and your business the most good. These will be essential to the foundation of the ideal condition I have in mind. I do not want a single town in the United States where there is a Rexall store to be without that foundation which is required for a tremendous publicity campaign for you and your stores.

The Egyptians may have built the first pyramids, but Liggett had his eyes on a new one.

Frustration was showing in a June letter less than three weeks later. "It looks to me as though 93 percent of our stockholders have failed to grasp what I am trying to do." So Liggett tried to help offering these ideas:

First—the existing stockholders still did not realize the value of having influential people in town also being stockholders.

Second—the individual stockholders do not seem to realize the profits to be gained by expansion of the stockholder base.

Third—the individual stockholder feels inadequate to the task of approaching potential stock buyers.

The rest of the message to the Pardners was filled with tips on how to correct these problems. In a related letter, Liggett referred to the Boot's organization (England), asking the rhetorical question, "Can you see the effect of having, as Boot's has, between 700 and 800 stockholders surrounding each of his stores?"

By July of the same year, Liggett's Dear Pardner letter acknowledged the terrible financial loss he had suffered, as described in Chapter 1. His optimism, however, seemed undiminished. In all capital letters he affirmed, "THE UNITED DRUG COMPANY IS AS SOUND AS A NUT, AND SO IS LIGGETT'S INTERNATIONAL."

Although he had personally "come to grief," he advised:

> [U]nless you owe money on your stocks and are forced to, don't sell a share of our stock. . . . [Y]ou are riding in the saddle; I am leading the horse, and I propose to continue to do so irrespective of what the Stock Market may do to my personal affairs.

It was an impassioned letter, too long to reproduce here, but he recounted his efforts to protect the stock at the expense of his own fortune. He refused any pessimism, and his final sentence goes a long way toward explaining what later happened:

> If this letter seems to you to be overly intimate, please realize that I feel an intimacy with you that has allowed me to recite to you my personal affairs in a manner that I would naturally like to keep back.

His New Year's letter in 1922 was typical. "WELCOME—1922! WE ARE READY FOR YOU!" And he was. Thanks to the support of his stockholders his affairs were already out of trusteeship and United was, by his account, in the best financial position since 1917.

In the next New Year's letter, it was time for a scolding. Some 28 out of every 100 stockholders were on the "no credit" list and 70 percent would not answer letters of inquiry. Typical of Liggett, he used his own experience in a plea for cooperation:

> To any of you who may be in the No Credit class, let me say that from personal experience only a short time ago I found that the strongest way to establish credit is to—

PUT YOUR CARDS ON THE TABLE.

We can help a good many of these twenty-eight percent to get off the No Credit list if they will only tell us why it is that they cannot pay their bills. I am going to make a personal effort this year to help these fellows, and I have asked the Credit Department to have all these problems that are of a serious nature brought to me. It may be embarrassing to write about one's financial affairs, but Boys, IT'S THE THING TO DO. *I KNOW!* Won't you let me try to help you as you helped me?

In June 1923, even though he had warned stockholders he would be in England for the summer, Liggett found time to write from Nottingham. It was a geography and cultural lesson that certainly was news to most of the readers. The biggest news, without going into financial detail, was that Liggett's International, all of whose voting stock was owned by United, had traded a quarter interest in Boot's for a one-seventh interest in United—and that United was debt free.

In October 1924, three years after the formation of the Rexall Loyalty Trust Fund to help Liggett out of his financial troubles, he was able to tell his Pardners that it was now possible to pay off in full and with interest the money raised. Surely this must have been one of his favorite Dear Pardner letters.

Chapter 3

The Sense of Family and Its Effects: Rexall Retirees Speak

The subtitle of Studs Terkel's (1972) remarkable book *Working* is *People Talk About What They Do All Day and How They Feel About What They Do.* That is what this chapter is about.

In Chapter 2, we saw how hard Liggett tried to build the Rexall "family." He referred to them as Pardners but often addressed them (not in a demeaning way) as his thousands of children. Sometimes he had to scold, but never severely. Mostly he offered opportunities and advice intended to help his children do well.

As this is being written, in 2004, more than seventy Rexall retirees are members of The Rexall Retirees Club. Not all, or even most, knew Liggett, but it is clear from their comments that a family spirit had been spawned in the company and that it survives.

This chapter consists primarily of quotations from conversations and correspondence with former Rexall employees. I did not hear from everyone, but I believe what follows captures the flavor of how the retirees feel—and they feel deeply, although they do not always agree.

The names of all of these respondents appear in the acknowledgments, but the quotes are not personally attributed. Many anticipate materials in later chapters. What I have tried to supply is the range of opinions among "insiders" about what happened to Rexall. So, let us begin with the first reminiscence:

> As I perceived it, we were where the *people* were when Rexall was strong, and then we let the people go to Kmart and Wal-Mart. We weren't where the people were. The corner drugstore left, and that's where we were. We didn't go into mass merchandising as we should have, probably. . . .

[In response to my comment that I still see Rexall signs around] There are still some places. We identified the corner drugstore, and then we didn't make our franchise as strong as, say, McDonald's. We kept lowering our standards and trying to get more outlets, I guess. I don't know. . . .

[Commenting on today's graduating pharmacists as a factor] Another thing that changed the retail drug business was having the fellows [*sic,* mostly female today] go through to get doctor of pharmacy [degrees], and that took the merchandising out of it. . . .

We were a great, great company. . . .

[But] Mr. Dart wasn't sure he wanted to put in all the money that was necessary to bring the company up to snuff, so to speak. We were a look-back-and-see-what-we-did-last-year kind of thing. (PC 32)[1]

Another respondent (PC 33) had sixty-five years with the company. He had met Liggett early in his career and, not knowing his identity, denied him access to certain parts of the plant on orders from his boss. Liggett, when he found out the facts, was high in his praise of this young man who knew how to follow orders.

One respondent (PC 64) started with Rexall in junior high school, sold Super Plenamins door-to-door, and was ultimately hired into a sales position by then President John Bowles. He found Justin Dart to be a "far-sighted man," a true "industrialist." He thought the Tupperware acquisition was a "stroke of genius"—a view not shared by all Rexall alumni.

Another respondent (PC 19), with thirty-plus years in the various Rexall-related operations, was forthcoming with his comments, which are quite revealing:

Rexall was a very, very good company for whom to work. I never had a problem going to the office, as something new happened every day. I do not know what wrongdoing you had to do in order to be discharged. They even hired the disabled long before it became the thing to do.

Rexall Family Druggists were numerous across the country. I did not have the privilege of knowing all of them. The ones I did were as much a part of the *Rexall Family* [emphasis added] as the employees.

One-Cent Sales were held twice a year. I looked forward to them much like Christmas.

Many people blame the executives who came after the company was sold for its demise. I agree that some contributed. Rexall was bought by Ross-Hall, and they had no experience with employees or unions. We were never informed what their business was. . . .

I feel Justin Dart was the real culprit. Rather than investing Rexall's profits back into our business, he used it to purchase other companies. One goal in his life was to have his name well-known. Ironically, when he merged with Kraft (known as Dart-Kraft), he thought his name would go on forever. I wonder what he would think now that the only thing his name is known for is being part of Reagan's Kitchen Cabinet, and that too is fading. . . .

[And in a very insightful comment] After the purchase by Ross-Hall, those in charge were concerned that large shopping centers and discount stores would replace the freestanding Rexall stores, and we began to neglect them. Look what Walgreens has done with their freestanding stores!

With her permission, I now will summarize some of the remarks of Norma Bowles, widow of John Bowles, former president of Rexall. She is clearly proud of her late husband's career with Rexall, recalling that he was recruited from his native North Carolina to California by Justin Dart, who was just setting up the new headquarters there. Dart thought that California would be a more pleasant environment for his executives.

By her account, her husband was a natural salesman and sales trainer. He taught that *resale* was more important than the first sale. He loved the "poppa and momma" druggists who were typical of Rexall franchises of the times. He treated his sales staff and their customers as "family," arranging for pictures in the home office of any visiting Rexallite. When he scheduled a sales meeting over the Easter holiday, he arranged to have an Easter bonnet delivered to the wife of each salesman who was away, and he also arranged for wives' luncheons during the sales meetings.

A major political coup to show free enterprise in action was John Bowles' arrangement with the U.S. Department of labor to install a model of a Rexall Drug Store at the Polish Trade Fair in Poznan, Poland, in 1960. John and his wife, Norma, were the mama and papa druggists chosen by Luther Hodges, then Secretary of Labor, to show Communists behind the Iron Curtain who visited the drugstore that free enterprise could provide a greater variety of goods at less cost than merchandise being sold in their apoteka. The President Eisenhower People-to-People Award was presented to the Bowles at the White House that year and Rexall could take a bow for for penetrating the Iron Curtain and communist thinking about free enterprise.

One respondent (PC 52) had been with the company in one form or another for forty-four years. In talking of his long experience in sales he said, "It was a lot of fun." As a sort of justification for the sale of Rexall to Ross-Hall in 1977 he noted:

> Actually the program as it was designed in its heyday was at that point [when it was sold] losing its *punch,* because in the 1940s and 1950s and 1960s it started losing its appeal. We had some of the strongest franchise stores in the country; only the best promoters would take the Rexall franchise, and that's the only ones to whom we would grant the franchise.

The respondent noted that competition changed (chains, discounters) and fair trade was gone. Rexall's sales force was reduced from 250 to 100 after the sale to Ross-Hall and he recounted the sale "for a song" after bankruptcy in 1985 to the company that became Rexall Sundown.

He recalled that "Rexall promotions were unequaled" in the 1950s:

> There was nothing on the face of the earth to equal [the One-Cent Sale]. Everyone knew about these sales. The name Rexall was so well-known. People knew the store was independently owned, but it appeared to be a national chain, which in essence it was.

When the company became Rexall Sundown, there were no longer any "Rexallites," although they were told they could keep their signs. According to another respondent:

> There were some very loyal people in the heyday; if Rexall had it, they bought it there instead of another store. We had a lot of over-the-counter stuff with the Rexall name on it, and when we sold the franchise to someone, we told them they could sell this as [their] label. That was working so well, Rexall started making its own cosmetics, paper towels, heating pads, etc., and if they could buy from Rexall, they would buy it. . . .

> My father's hangout was the local Rexall store. . . . Because of this friend, the Rexall pharmacist, I always wanted to be a "druggist." I would fill my Radio Flyer wagon with bottles and containers and act out dispensing medicine to my cats and dogs (PC 51).

Unfortunately, he never got to be a druggist. He did attend two years of pharmacy school but was asked to drop out temporarily because of the shortage of pharmacists to teach classes during the war. A promise to finance his education never came to pass, but he did stay in the drug business and with that store.

> We were one of the better Rexall stores in the state. One of the things we would look forward to were the One-Cent Sales. Later we were involved with their monthly sales promotions. We would attend various Rexall Club meetings, attend the Christmas shows to purchase Christmas goods. Of course, we featured Cara-Nome cosmetics, and Stag products for men.
>
> The year after the owners purchased the store, we bought a second store, a Walgreen Agency store. Of course, we threw Walgreens out the door and stocked the new acquisition with Rexall products. I was installed as a partner in the ownership of the two stores. We would go all-out with the Rexall sales, piling products in case stacks, placing signs on all of the windows, and promoting the sales with vigor.
>
> We caught one of the partners stealing funds and kicked him out of the partnership. Shortly after that, the remaining partner died, leaving me with all of the indebtedness and not being a Registered Pharmacist, I sold the stores. . . .
>
> I started working for Rexall as a rep for accounts in the St. Louis area. At that time, Rexall was the dominating force in the retail drug field. As the time passed, everything looked good.

Things [then] began to turn sour. Justin Dart lost interest in the drugstore field and sold the company to some investors who knew nothing about the drugstore business. After that sale, the wheels started to come off of the company. Instead of trying to be happy with our solid base of independent stores, Rexall started to expand into areas that were not to the liking of our independent stores. The independent store owners became angry when Rexall went into Wal-Mart and supermarkets, and the independent stores started to cancel their franchises.

In addition to expanding the Rexall products into other outlets, they started to pare the lines, which also irritated the independent stores even more. The sales force was down to just a few sales reps calling on "mass merchandisers" and "brokers." For the most part, these food brokers knew nothing about the drugstore business and could care less about selling a few hundred dollars of Rexall products when they could sell truckloads of other products.

[In] January 1982, I was terminated from Rexall, along with many other sales reps who had years of experience, and they went with a bunch of young reps who could not sell the Rexall concept, thus the final *gasp*—bankruptcy.

It broke my heart to see the company that I had decided to cast my future with go down the tube, so to speak. I think that the downfall of the company was not to fulfill the needs of the 10,000 stores who supported Rexall for years. Rexall had been a large family of stores with like needs and by not fulfilling these needs, Rexall became expendable, thus the end of an era.

One respondent (PC 40) described the span of his Rexall career: "I began working in a Rexall drugstore when I was fifteen years old; that adds up to sixty-one years ago in 1942. After being discharged from the Navy, I worked there before and after I attended college." Another respondent summed up his experiences with Rexall:

I began my career with Rexall in July 1957 in Columbus, Ohio.... The big dance was over in 1982 and I was fifty-five years old. I took a month off, then went to work for a local wholesaler. I then really understood what superior training we had with Rexall. In my seven years with the wholesaler, I did their advertising program, buying, worked on the road part time, and opened a new area for them. I believed in the idea that new business was the life blood of any company, unlike many in Rexall, who just filled basements and garages with Rexall merchandise.

I think the greatest thing we had was the camaraderie of our sales force and the relationship we formed between our partners. (The Rexall Druggist, as Louis K. Liggett, our founder, so aptly coined it.)

If you think about it, we had a group of good guys back from the second World War, a part of Tom Brokaw's greatest generation, eager to succeed and make it happen. As we use to say, "Just don't stand there, sell something."

We also had Justin Dart, a real sharp president, who thank goodness had the foresight during the golden years of pharmacy, when we made nothing but money, to use it wisely. He formed a larger company with a lot of good smaller companies into Dart Industries.

Rexall was more than just a company; it was a religion of sorts, with a lot of good, loyal people. We had lots of fun at meetings and Christmas gift shows and formed lasting relationships. I still have lunch once a month with a retired Rexall druggist. I talk on the phone and e-mail with several Rexall salesmen.

Rexall premiered many ideas that I still see being used in retailing today. For example: The Rexall One-Cent Sale, I see that concept in many retail outlets.

The franchise idea itself—Rexall was the first franchiser in America. Look at all the franchisers today. We made our own goods. How many retailers do I see using that concept, from Wal-Mart, the biggest with their Equate line of health and beauty aids, to the food chains with their own label? Money-back guarantees on all Rexall products, fully guaranteed to the consumer, was another first. Quality—our generic pharmaceuticals were used by the Philadelphia College of Pharmacy, a very prestigious operation.

What happened to Rexall? Well, I believe we were just a victim of the changing times in retailing. Our business was with the small, independent drugstores across America and when the big word *discount* appeared on the scene, the stores began to disappear.

Commenting on franchise relationships, one respondent noted:

Charlie Walgreen was one of the first franchisers. He and Louie Liggett, our owner, had a misunderstanding and he told Mr. Liggett, "I'll do the same as you," and he started his Walgreen franchises. . . .
I couldn't believe the demise of Rexall, but the new owners had no firm commitment to the franchisees. They were not good businesspeople. It was not [the fault of] Justin Dart! (PC 20)

One respondent (PC 31), in praise of Dart, said, "I had a wonderful corporate life with Justin Dart for nearly thirty years, and he transformed the business into a respected and highly successful conglomerate company before the merger with Kraft."

Quality leadership led some respondents to view Rexall as an extended family:

During my years with this company, the Rexall program was one of the few available to the independent pharmacy. This program gave the independent national recognition, a line of exclusive products under the Rexall label, and preplanned promotions throughout the year. The most popular of the promotions was the semiannual and famous One-Cent Sale. In years past, discounting was not offered in drugstores, and the One-Cent Sale was the first to offer a discount to the consumer. Many customers would buy products like shave cream, mouthwash, toothpaste, etc., by the case because they recognized the savings that were not available otherwise. . . .
In years past the Rexall drugstore was highly recognized in most towns and communities. At one time, they numbered over 10,000 stores nationally. Consumers not only thought of the Rexall store as a source for prescriptions and other health needs, but many of them had soda fountains. Friends would meet there to visit and enjoy their favorite refreshments. I can still remember buying an ice cream cone at the Rexall in my hometown for a nickel.

Over the years Rexall became somewhat like a big family and I still have co-workers and Rexallites that are good friends.

As we know, everything changes with time. As large chain drugstores and mammoth discount stores moved in, the role of the neighborhood drugstore diminished. This had its effects on Rexall as well, and the rest is history. The villain was mainly a change in time and circumstances. (PC 12)

Another respondent described the glory and decline of Rexall:

It was a great privilege to work under the great personality and motivational JOHN BOWLES, who not only inspired the entire sales force to better sales but traveled over the entire country, visiting Rexall franchised drugstores in the large cities down to the smallest hamlets. John was, indeed, "MR. REXALL" to Rexallites and salespeople alike, and the terrific impact he made on everyone that he met was the glue that made Rexall and the independent Rexall drugstores the strongest retail factor in the country. He was a great man, and to all the Rexall drugstores he was, indeed, the driving force of a great company. . . .

A few years later Justin Dart sold the Rexall Division to a group who were dedicated to the ultimate demise of a drugstore franchise that was so important to the independent druggist and whose employees were such great contributors to the success of the Rexall Drug Company. Sadly enough, the sale of the Rexall Drug Company was the forerunner of the demise of the independent drugstore.

Rexall's One-Cent Sale was the first great sales event for Rexall drugstores, and the impact on their sales and on the sales of each Rexall sales representative was something to behold.

It was a very sad day, indeed, when Justin Dart disposed of the Rexall Drug Company, and, again, not only did loyal employees of the company suffer as a result, but also the Rexall drugstores ceased to be the strong retailers that they were. Times have changed, of course, but, today, Mr. and Mrs. Consumer cannot drive from state to state looking for that familiar Rexall sign, looking for the products and prices that they had known [and] were so loyal to over the years. A very sad day took place when Rexall was no longer a force in the marketplace.

Today there is a "new" Rexall—who purchased the Rexall Drug Company from the corporation that bought the firm from Dart. However, there is no comparison with the great Rexall Drug Company that we knew and loved. . . .

Rexall drugstores [and their operators] became an integral part of Rexall itself. They attended Rexall sales meetings; they had Rexall sales representatives conduct frequent in-store sales meetings, which greatly contributed to making their employees better salespeople, with more knowledge of Rexall products and the Rexall signs [all] over the country, with ten thousand Rexall franchisees, served as a beacon to the travelers and reminded them of the great products they had purchased from their hometown Rexall drugstore. . . .

Yes, Rexall was, indeed, a great company—one that inspired loyalties between Rexall salesmen, Rexall employees, and Rexall drugstores—a gone, but not forgotten, wonderful chapter in the history of drugstore retailing. (PC 6)

The following respondent reflected on the pros and cons of the Rexall era:

Having worked for one of the top Rexall stores in the country, I had a great working knowledge of merchandise, sales, promotions, etc. For the last few years of employment, I bought, stocked, and sold all Rexall products; attended conventions, etc.; and had the privilege of meeting Joe Galvin, the chairman of the board. I also had the privilege of meeting Phil Harris and Alice Faye.

Rexall was the best thing that ever happened to independent drugstores, and made the big difference in profits. Over the years, I called on and worked with hundreds of drugstores!

[The] One-Cent Sale was one of the biggest promotions, and certainly a great part of Americana. [Of] the two things that killed the One-Cent Sale, [one] was the government saying we couldn't advertise this way because the items were being discounted and were no longer a true two for one. The number two reason was management was not able to come up with a new format to make the government happy.

The real villain in the demise of Rexall was the age of management! As the management aged and continued to run the company, they were more interested in retaining a status quo for retirement. Therefore, for years they continued to run the same promotions, repeating what had been unsuccessful in the past. Druggists got tired of simply buying more merchandise and dropped most promotions.

When Rexall stopped earning profits commensurate with the other divisions of Dart Industries, it became apparent that Rexall was in its waning years. Rexall merely survived for a few years, salesmen and managers were reduced in numbers, services were discontinued, and a general lack of management care resulted in the decision [of the company] finally being sold and subsequently disbanded.

The first time that Rexall was sold (to Commonwealth, United, which was [suspected of being] mafia owned, and the sale stopped by the Federal Government) was when I decided that the end was coming and started looking for a business to buy. [This sale was not completed.] (PC 5)

A widow of a man who, by her account, "was Rexall for thirty-eight years" made these comments:

My feelings over those years were a loyalty to Rexall also. It was a company to be proud of and we were. It was after Justin Dart became president and was busy forming his Dart Industries that it was evident Rexall was not his prime interest. Then John Bowles came on the scene, more obvious disinterest in the company, more [interest] in the title he held. The company was sold to people not interested in restoring what was lost, but just an investment. We had several presidents whose interest was not in Rexall.

While the company was healthy, there was good competition between representatives to keep their territory first in sales. The One-Cent Sales were always good, with special promotions included, such as goldfish and the bowl—I'm not sure as a giveaway or a low price. Christmas shows in July always brought a lot of the druggists in to purchase their Christmas merchandise. These were hard work but seemed to do the job. (PC 65)

Another respondent grew up with Rexall:

> I was born in a Rexall family. The year of my birth (1936) my father purchased the store from my aunt. I still have a copy of that pink franchise. I started to work in the store at age fourteen and quickly learned how much work it took to set the One-Cent Sale and the Rexall PM programs. One sale that was always successful was the "goldfish" promotion. My job was to put two goldfish in the bowl with seaweed and chips and build a display without making a mess. My father was a true Rexallite, one that ran all sales and promotions one hundred percent, circulars included, and sold a lot of merchandise. Many of the salesmen I knew then, and later on in my career, could convince an account to rent a garage and stock up on Mi31, Klenzo, alcohol, etc., that many would think should last for years, but only took a short time to sell.
>
> I worked part-time until I joined the Navy after graduating from high school. I was hired by Rexall when I was twenty-four years old. At that time most new trainees came from Rexall drugstores. My first territory was southern Ohio, Kentucky, and West Virginia. Many of the accounts in that area were part of the original forty agents set up by Louis Liggett, called the United Drug Company. Rexall had many ideas that were before their time—ideas that competitors tried to put down but used after Rexall was gone. . . .
>
> What happened to Rexall? *My opinion [is that] it started when Rexall gave franchises to the chain stores*, especially when the chain had stores next to good independents. In Ohio, it was Gray's Drug of Cleveland [later Revco now CVS]. They put thousands of dollars of merchandise in stores under a guarantee sale.
>
> It did not take Gray's long to figure out that they could produce their own private-label merchandise, which they did and [then] promptly sent all Rexall merchandise back to the Columbus warehouse. Most of this merchandise was not resalable. It took Rexall a few years to get over that before insulting the Rexallite again by putting their merchandise into wholesalers who sold to everyone (Bergen in California). It didn't take Bergen (long) to take control!
>
> Justin Dart was a good businessman. He knew he could make more in real estate, Tupperware, and other ventures than in the

drug business. That is why he "spun off" that part of Dart Industries. . . .

As a Rexall representative, I loved it! I have many memories from many conventions. I saw a lot of cities I would not have visited if it hadn't been for these meetings. As a Rexall rep, you learned and you were a merchandiser. (PC 23)

A number of respondents speculated on Rexall's demise:

I guess it began about 1978, when Dart finally sold it to the holding company, and during that period of time, in 1980, I moved into the home office in marketing. The decision was made to go open market for twofold reasons. Drop the OTCs [over-the-counter drugs] because the vitamins were more profitable and easier to make. And the OTCs because the equipment was not state of the art, and it got to where it was too expensive to make stuff and a lot more problems to pass the muster as far as the FDA [Food and Drug Administration], etc. If you get the FDA out of there on the drug end of it and deal with them on the supplement end of it, it's a whole different story. The equipment for the vitamins was much better. The reality was that the independent drugstore was waning, and you could only have one per little town, and the growth was not there, and in reality that was true. It happened all at one time, at the worst economic time around. Inflation was twenty percent and interest rates were twenty percent, so the people did not have the money to back it up, or didn't want to back it up, so it basically sunk. It was bad management and what have you—good thinking not brought to fruition—and when it got down to the point where there was nothing left, that's when the sale went through. (PC 43)

I don't think Justin Dart wanted to be associated with Rexall Drug anymore. He wanted to divorce himself from any relationship. He had no interest in making Rexall a successful company. I think most people who worked for Rexall used to think very highly of Justin Dart, and I totally changed my opinion about Justin Dart when I was at [headquarters]. I think he was selfish and self-gratifying. Why he let such a great company go down the drain, I don't know. (PC 42)

The respondent stated that both distributors and manufacturing facilities were antiquated. I told him that another retiree had said that when Rexall went into distribution instead of what they were doing it was the death knell. His answer:

> I'm not sure that was the death of it. Their own products were very limited. Most companies can make a living with five products. Rexall had over six hundred products. Why not take advantage of the fact that you have all these stores and they are going to buy from you? . . . Independent pharmacy was at the crossroads at that point, and franchising was about their only hope, and they lost it. Independent pharmacies had big chains like Rexall, and then they didn't have it anymore. . . .
>
> [Rexall] was the most wonderful name in the drug business. Most of their products were great; their packaging was terrible. . . . For the Rexall products, they were always ugly. (PC 42)

When I asked another retiree if he agreed with the opinion expressed that Dart got tired of the drug business and didn't pay enough attention to it, he responded in the affirmative:

> What you hear is true—that when Tupperware and West Bend were making money, and Rexall was just barely making money, [Dart] totally lost interest in it, so the advertising was cut and the One-Cent Sale lasted longer than it should have. After fair trade went out that killed the One-Cent Sale. All of these things put together with management had to do with it.
>
> It's an amazing story because there is nothing like it. It was doing so much good for independent pharmacists . . . it should have stayed and would have made a really big difference. . . . You went to a Rexall convention and it was just like a family reunion. (PC 8)

When asked what happened to Rexall, one respondent commented:

> We who worked for Rexall have discussed it many times. I think it was Justin Dart (you probably know his background). He married Charles Walgreen's daughter and was active in the Walgreens company for many years. When he became president of Rexall, I think he took hold of it and did some good things. I

don't think he ever envisioned a Rexall Drug Company as big as Walgreens today and as successful as Walgreens. I think he thought of it in his mind as small druggists that we were dealing with, and that was the maximum we could do. I don't think he ever liked the drug business that much because he branched off into other things like Tupperware. . . .

There could have been some survival of druggists in this area and others. As you know, it metamorphosed into these large pharmacies, chain pharmacies, and I think a lot of that is due to the fact that the pharmacists in the profession were not really organized either. [They are not called "independent" for no reason.]

We had a love-hate relationship with them. We were to talk to them about remaining in business and making their businesses stronger, and of course a lot of them just go along with the program. I would go into stores oftentimes and find our monthly sales kits just stacked [in the] back. They wouldn't put the signs up or anything. That was one of the great things we had back in those days to make the store look alive, and when people came in [to] have an item for sale that would attract them. . . .

One of the things that I think occurred was that some expert came in and told them to remove their [soda] fountains. They said they were losing money and it wasn't a good thing for their store. Pull the fountain out and fill it up with shelves. I think that was a bad thing in many small towns because it was almost a focal point for the people to come in, at least on Saturday night, and have a soda. . . .

I think when Justin Dart decided to get into other things, the company was neglected. And then when we knew that we couldn't retain our business with ten thousand small drugstores, they got into selling through the wholesalers, etc., and that was kind of botched up, and it just went from one bad thing to another. I think they hired a lot of people within the Rexall Drug Company who didn't grow up in the drug business like you and I did. I think that makes a lot of difference. Finally they just got down to hiring hatchet men to get rid of all of us, and it went from bad to worse.

> Rexall was one of the companies where they just loved it
> when a Rexall salesman called on them, and you felt like you
> were part of a family. (PC 38)

Another respondent had this to say:

> Dart had lost interest in the retail drug business. That was the big
> thing. Even having grown up "in the drug industry," he had a
> bigger vision, at least in his mind. I'm not criticizing him. He
> was a very smart man. He did a lot for Rexall. He put in a retire-
> ment plan, which was excellent.
>
> In the early 1950s, Dart became a great Eisenhower sup-
> porter. He was a great Eisenhower campaigner. He asked the
> company for a three-month leave of absence, and after that was
> up, he'd ask for another three. And so, therefore, about three or
> four years this went on, and Rexall wasn't doing anything; it
> was just drifting, with no leadership. It had great people work-
> ing for it, and that's the thing that held it together. . . .
>
> I got to know one of the members of the board of Rexall, and I
> can't think of his name, but he represented the Life Saver indus-
> tries, and Life Saver industries was one of the biggest stockhold-
> ers in Rexall. The company drifted and drifted, and finally this
> gentleman I am talking about told me the board of directors had
> a meeting without Dart, and he was chosen to speak to Dart
> about this . . . to either "shit or get off the pot." Dart was very
> gracious about it and then he went back to work.
>
> One of the first things he did was to buy out Tupperware. He
> went back to work, but not in the retail drug business. Then he
> started Riker Laboratories. Rexall had a big factory there in St.
> Louis, so he went into other things like that. Then he brought in
> John Bowles. . . .
>
> We had conventions; the first one I went to was in Atlantic
> City; druggists came from all over the country. We went to great
> shows. One of my druggists said he wanted to talk to Dart. He
> got in the elevator with his newspapers and said, "I'll see you to-
> morrow."
>
> They had a Rexall convention on Cape Cod and the main
> speaker was to be Calvin Coolidge. He was out on the presiden-
> tial yacht off the coast and they had this terrible rainstorm. Fi-
> nally he came ashore, and the Rexall person couldn't get the car

started; they found a car with the key in it, started it, and took off. They later said that was the first time the president rode in a stolen car. (PC 17)

I asked another Rexallite about the mechanics of the dissolution of the Rexall franchises. With 10,000 Rexall druggists, did Rexall simply say, "We're not doing this anymore?"

> Basically yes. It started somewhere between 1978 and 1980. I think Ross-Hall bought the company in 1978. It was just a holding company. One guy . . . was in charge of it all. You won't be able to find out anything about it. He had in years past some kind of Rexall association as a drugstore franchise or something. He had kind of a love for the company. I am trying to remember. I am pretty sure that [ending of franchises] happened after Ross-Hall bought it. I don't know if the idea came from there or if the idea was already in the works before that happened. The idea was that the independent drugstore is on its way [out] and it's not going to go up again. And you just can't tie yourself to that, and so we had to go open market. What they did . . . they came through and they played a little game on it. They had a little sign, kind of a release contract, and it wasn't a franchise. It was an agreement to continue carrying Rexall products . . . something like that. But basically what they were trying to do was eliminate the contract. (PC 43)

Rexall signs had always been a major part of the drugstore facade, and at one point, Ross-Hall (or another company) instructed pharmacists to take them down. Then they began reimbursing pharmacists for major repairs, so they decided the signs could stay up but they weren't paying for that. I presented this to one Rexallite (PC 43), who replied:

> To my knowledge that's true. They tested the waters, but basically they decided it wasn't worth the fight to do that. I was never asked to go and tell the stores to take down the signs. The way the piece of paper [which replaced the contract] read was pretty benign. It was very well written. Ninety percent of those signs were bought and paid for by the retailer. They kept saying

that we had a right to tell them to take down the signs, but they weren't going to fight any battles. They said they would just eventually go away, which they almost all have.

It was my good fortune to have an opportunity for in-person interviews with two Rexall retirees (PCs 19 and 71) simultaneously. This fascinating interchange follows:

SMITH: Who do you think was the villain?

PC 71: Ross-Hall. But if they hadn't put the company up for sale, Ross-Hall wouldn't have been there to buy it.

SMITH: Who was that?

PC 19: Well, you are going back to Dart. I don't blame Dart for what he did.

PC 71: Well, of course he built it, but then knocked it down. What does that say?

PC 19: Justin Dart took a company like Rexall and he built an empire, but the only thing he didn't do was put money back into it. He was in the middle of the thing.

PC 71: He sold the mother company off, which was unheard of. Rexall was the fat cow, the mother, and he sold it off to buy other companies.

PC 19: He was a hero to the stockholders, but we think he is a villain, because he just threw us out to the dogs.

SMITH: [Distribution question] Was there ever any effort to put together a co-op toward the end to keep it going?

PC 71: That's what they did when they started closing up our distribution centers. They all went to this private distribution center. That's what started Rexall to begin with. By that time all the druggists were very unhappy with Rexall.

SMITH: I was thinking that if enough of them got together and put together a corporation, they could buy it out, keep the Rexall name, and keep it going.

PC 71: Later on down the road Rexall druggists were not loyal to the name.

PC 19: Why would they be? We were so nasty to them.

Here is a conversation with a final, but very important respondent:

SMITH: You weren't there when Ross Hall did the acquisition, is that correct?

PC 68: Yes, I was there when they did the acquisition on January 7, 1977, I think. I had a heart attack in 1980, and I essentially was out of the picture from that period on and moved out to California.

SMITH: Who was the owner when Ross-Hall made the acquisition?

PC 68: Rexall was a part of Dart's organization at that time. . . . we were Dart Industries, and we were the mother company of a string of acquisitions that Justin Dart made. Tupperware and all those.

SMITH: Exactly. I really am trying to get a handle on who Ross-Hall is.

PC 68: I wish that I could tell you that because Ross-Hall was just a name that was a group of investors. Ross-Hall disappeared when Rexall disappeared, as far as I can determine, and what was left of Rexall was sold to a group of people from Florida.

SMITH: Right. Rexall Sundown.

PC 68: And who they were I have no idea.

SMITH: Who were the principals, if you can tell me, of Ross-Hall? What I have been told is that they were a holding company, and the only name I have is someone named Brown.

PC 68: Bill Brown was one of the principal people with Ross-Hall. . . .

SMITH: How long were you with Rexall in one form or another?

PC 68: I joined Rexall in 1947 and went until 1980—about thirty-five years, my whole career. And in those days, when I joined the company as a sales representative, it was kind of expected that you would stay with the company all your life.

SMITH: That's what I am getting. . . . There was a great sense of family, and everybody is there to stay.

PC 68: Yes, there was a great familial feeling, and it was "Mother" Rexall almost. . . . Anyway, the company was sold in 1977, and it had been no secret that the company was up for sale. It always made money, but it was stable . . . it didn't progress, making the amount of money that Justin Dart wanted to make on his investment. So he sort of traded companies and bought and sold them almost as if you and I would go out and buy and sell a dozen eggs. . . .

He was a brilliant man. I admire and respect him. Of course he is dead now.

SMITH: I was told . . . by one of my correspondents on the phone that he blamed [one person] for the dissolution of Rexall—that he had gone to Ross-Hall and said, "I'm going to eliminate the sales force and save you a lot of money if you will just make me president." Does that make any sense to you?

PC 68: It does and it doesn't. [He] was kind of a wild guy. He set up a telephone calling system with Rexall called "Rexcall," and it was actually fairly successful—for direct selling. At one time, shortly after I took over about 1972, we had about two hundred twenty salesmen and about fifteen districts. And by going to the telephone, we cut down a lot of routine reordering and speeded up the system, so I suppose if it were now it would have become computerized, as they all have. . . .

I think anybody in the business could see the handwriting on the wall. The basic reason is that the independent drugstore was dead. There were ten thousand Rexall drugstores, but they were not all great stores. And with the supermarkets going into pharmacies, the handwriting was on the wall that the independent druggist living on what he did up front was a mastodon. . . .

SMITH: What percentage would you put on the end of Rexall as a major franchise organization protecting the independent druggist as a franchisee? How much of it was because the franchisee wasn't doing the job, and how much of it was because the corporation had changed its policy, was selling to wholesalers and to chains, etc.?

PC 68: I think you might find some of each. Do you remember the One-Cent Sale? We had a cease and desist order from the Federal Trade Commission. Almost fifty percent of our business was done on billing for those two events for the year. And of course we couldn't use that idea of two for the price of one plus a penny, because we couldn't prove that every store had the same basic price. When fair trade was going, NARD [National Association of Retail Druggists] was the biggest proponent of that—they lost, of course. That kind of let the horse out of the barn as far as Rexall was concerned. . . .

SMITH: Do you know any place where I can find out more about the Ross-Hall group? They weren't publically held, I know that, and it just seems almost impossible to get a line on who they were. Are you telling me that was just a name for the company and had nothing to do with the principals?

PC 68: I think it was a name. They were financial people and not marketing people. I have never seen that name, Ross-Hall Corporation, used anywhere except with Rexall acquisitions. . . .

The problem with the Ross-Hall group was underfinancing. They were given a good deal by Justin Dart, and then when it came to running the business and you need money for inventory, equipment, people, and all of those things, that's another question. My opinion is that they were underfinanced, because they sold off the building on Kingshighway where the manufacturing was done, and our office was there. In order to raise money, they used leverage on everything, including selling the building and leasing it back, which is the traditional thing to do, but eventually the bank called in their note, and I think they were underfinanced.

SMITH: One respondent said that they only bought it as a tax loss in the first place.

PC 68: That makes sense, because they had other ventures which I wasn't privy to. They had them overseas and in this country, too. England, Japan, South Africa, etc.

What can be discerned from this small and not necessarily representative sample of opinions? (It would have been wonderful to hear from a few hundred of those Rexall family druggists.) Here are some points to consider:

- The consensus is that Rexall was a great company.
- A sense of "family" existed among Rexall employees.
- The Rexall denouement created a sense of great loss.
- Liggett laid a foundation based on genius and personal force.
- The independent druggist benefited greatly from the Rexall concept and lost much when the franchise aspect was killed. (Whether the independent was doomed anyway is moot.)
- Justin Dart was a giant figure who simply "moved on" to projects other than the drug business. (Whether hero or villain depends upon to whom you are talking.)

PART II:
MARKETING REXALL

Chapter 4

The Genius of Rexall Product

In Part II we use a framework based on the well-known four Ps of marketing. Each of these, with the definitions I used in my 1991 textbook, *Pharmaceutical Marketing: Strategy and Cases,*[1] follows:

1. *Product:* The benefits and positive results that markets derive out of doing business with your company using the products you offer in the way that you offer them
2. *Price:* The total cost components that customers must bear in order to use the products offered
3. *Place:* The distribution channels and physical distribution practices that make it possible, easy, or difficult to use the products
4. *Promotion:* What and how markets are informed of the firm's product, price, and place

It should be obvious that the four Ps are interrelated, and that was the case with Rexall, as shall be demonstrated in this and the following three chapters.

PRODUCT MERCHANDISING

The reader is reminded of the words of the Rexall Family Druggist in the preface: that the "2,000 or more products made by the Rexall Drug Company . . . are as fine and pure and dependable as science can make them." What a terrific statement!

Still, two thousand products from a company that started in an empty building with *no* products? That's quite a product story. Indeed, the question (if there ever *were* any questions) in Liggett's mind should have been, "What do we start with?"

Based on one of his Dear Pardner letters, the first product was Dyspepsia Cure, and this product, along with cleverly introducing the Rexall name to the public, formed the basis for Liggett's first promotion to the public. Almost immediately he also began producing *candy* in the basement of his newly acquired Boston facility.

It should be remembered that Liggett had two kinds of "customers" for his products: (1) stockholders and franchisees and the general public. This provides but one example of the essential interaction of the four Ps. United Drug needed to produce quality products in which the druggists not only had faith but also would vigorously recommend to their customers—so-called "push" promotion. Then it was also necessary, through promotion to the general public, to convince them that Rexall products were as good as, or better than, those offered by their more familiar, brand-name competitors. Even if both of these efforts were successful, that success could be sustained only if United Drug "delivered the goods." Liggett was well aware of how fickle the public, and for that matter the druggists, could be.

From the outset Liggett insisted on the highest quality in production and hired the kind of people to make this happen. It is well to remember that when United Drug began production, and for many years thereafter, the quality of drug products was left to the manufacturer. No FDA inspector peered over the shoulder of the head of production. High-quality products were not just the right thing to do; they were good business.

It must be borne in mind that the effectiveness of many of the drug products extant during these early days was questionable. What is "dyspepsia" anyway? Is there really a "cure"? *Cure* tended to be more or less a euphemism for symptom relief, which of course increases the chances of repeat sales—a desirable characteristic in any product.

Clinical trials as we know them today were nonexistent, but quality control and other testing were very much a part of the United Drug policy. In 1906 the federal government did make its first, tentative steps into the regulation of the manufacture of drugs by passing the Pure Food and Drug Act, requiring the manufacturer to print on product labels all of the ingredients contained therein. This was no problem for United Drug, as that had been their policy since the company began production. It was, however, a problem for some of their competitors, who were either known to be or suspected of using some form of narcotics. (No wonder repeat sales were good!)

In 1909 United Drug Company of Canada was formed, only after another legal hurdle. An already established, though small, company there was using a Rexall trademark. (It would be interesting to know who coined the name there and when.) United finally bought the company and began the manufacture of Rexall Cherry Juice Cough Syrup and Mucutone, the latter being one of Rexall's most successful products.

In 1910, just seven years after the company started, a 140,000-square-foot laboratory was added to the original Boston facility—evidence of commitment to quality products and to developing new ones. More new products were being added to the line on a regular basis, often by acquisition or special arrangements with other companies. Certainly, not all new products were *drug* products, but they were all *drugstore* products. Examples include the following:

- Candy, of course, including the products of the Guth Chocolate Company
- Water (!), by a quid pro quo with the Ballardville Springs Water Company
- Cigars, as noted in Chapter 1
- Fire insurance—yes, fire insurance
- Soda fountain supplies, by purchase of the F. L. Daggett Company
- Stationery, through formation of the United Stationery Company
- Rubber goods, through acquisition of Seamless Rubber Company
- Cotton goods, through purchase of the Absorbent Cotton Company
- Perfumes and toiletries, through agreement with the Hanson-Jacks Company
- Grape juice, which would become an important product during Prohibition, by acquiring Schule Pure Grape Juice

In 1919 a new product line was "invented." Prior to this Rexall had sold such remedies as castor oil, rubbing alcohol, Epsom salts, and cod liver oil in bulk for repackaging by the druggist. Rexall now began to prepackage these products in different and convenient sizes. The name chosen for this new line of products, "Puretest," was yet another stroke of genius, suggesting as it did just what both sets of customers wanted.

In 1928 major product-related events began to happen. Through a series of negotiations, United reached an agreement with Sterling Products. This resulted in a major addition to the product line. A partial list of the medications, household names all, to which United now had unlimited access included these:

- Danderine
- Cascarets
- Bayer Aspirin
- Phillips' Milk of Magnesia
- Midol

Again, the details of these corporate mating games are beyond the scope of this account, but the United/Sterling engagement allowed a joint *adventure,* resulting in the acquisition by the newly formed Drug, Inc. (United and Sterling), of the following products:

- Life Savers
- 3-In-1 Oil
- Fletcher's Castoria
- Caldwell's Syrup of Pepsin
- Scott's Emulsion
- Mum

Later that year the Vicks Chemical Company was taken over, bringing VapoRub and Vitalis into the product line.

It is important to understand that throughout this process of adding products by acquisition and merger, Rexall was busy developing products internally. In the course of the Tenth Annual Rexall Convention, held in St. Louis, President Liggett reported on Company progress. As reported in the October 12, 1914 issue of *Rexall Advantages,* Liggett noted:

> During the year . . . we have manufactured and sold 162,220,000 pills and tablets, all trademarked (with the name Rexall, of course);
> 221,540 pounds of talcum powder, representing over one million packages . . .
>
> 605,863 bottles of hair tonic;
> 182,176 pounds of cold cream;
> 161,490 pounds of ointments and salves;

343,848 packages of toothpaste;
9,211,390 cold tablets;
46,000,000 Orderlies [a laxative]—one for every other person in
the United States.

He continued with statistics on shipments of perfume, playing cards, pencils, fountain pens, chocolates, and fountain supplies and added: "Last but not least, we sold in the last eight weeks 1,500 alligators (live)." There seemed to be no end to the variety of products.

The same issue of *Rexall Ad-Vantages* offered special deals on Rexall goldfish. (It is not known if the Rexall logo was imprinted on each fish.) The fish, guaranteed to arrive live, were shipped in lots of 288 along with appropriate accessories. The druggists, to whom *Ad-Vantages* was directed, were urged to "offer these outfits FREE to purchasers of a 25 cent Rexall remedy and watch your sales jump."

What follows is a partial list of products being offered to Rexall druggists for sale to the public in 1913:

Rexall Liver Salts
Rexall Antiseptic Tooth Powder
Rexall Kidney Pills
Rexall Baby Cough Syrup
Rexall Beef, Wine and Iron Tonic
Rexall Blemish Soap
Rexall Carbolic Salve
Rexall Celery and Iron Tonic
Rexall Charcoal Tablets
Rexall Cherry Bark Cough Syrup
Rexall Cod Liver Oil Emulsion
Rexall Cold Tablets
Rexall Corn Solvent
Rexall Eczema Ointment
Rexall Eu-Zo-Mol
Rexall Foot Powder
Rexall Grippe Pills
Rexall Kidney Remedy
Rexall Laxative Syrup
Rexall Mentholine Balm
Rexall Pile Treatment
Rexall Rheumatic Remedy

Rexall Rubbing Oil
Rexall Sarsaparilla Tonic
Rexall Specific and Alternative Compound
Rexall Thymo Dentaline
Rexall Vegetable Compound
Rexall Vegetable Compound (Spanish)
Rexall Wine of Cod Liver Extract
Rexall Headache Wafers

Printed circulars describing each product were also for sale to the druggists. One such circular (intended to be distributed to customers) is reprinted here verbatim, as it speaks to the quality of Rexall products.

When you buy clothing or groceries, you insist upon quality—quality is the first consideration.

But do you always insist upon quality—do you always **get** quality—when you buy drugs?

*There is infinitely more reason why you should insist upon quality and make sure you **get** quality in buying drugs than in anything else you can buy.*

The liability of many drugs to deteriorate with age, or when improperly kept, and the deplorable tendency sometimes found in some druggists to buy drugs of inferior quality, because they feel sure that you, who are not a pharmacist, will not know the difference, makes the matter of buying drugs something that you should be very careful about.

We buy and sell only drugs of **tested quality, absolute purity,** and **full standard strength**—not through fear that you might find us out if we did otherwise, but because the store that always sells drugs that give satisfaction and yield the results expected of them is the one that will get and keep trade.

And then, there is something more than trade compensation to be derived from doing business right—*there is the satisfaction of doing right.*

Nor do the quality requirements at this store stop at drugs. They extend to every other line we carry, whether it be rubber goods, perfumery, stationery, bristle goods, no matter what—you are always sure of getting quality—and at right prices at **The Rexall Store**

Of course, all of these and many other Rexall products were for sale to and through only Rexall druggists.

A sense of product strategies and dynamics can be gained from the comparisons that follow. Looking thirty years ahead to 1943 (during World War II), we find a much more extensive list of Rexall products:[2]

A. B. C. Seltzer
Acid Dyspepsia Tablets
Aga-Rex (compound and plain)
Alternative Compound
Analgesic Balm
Analgesic Balm (greaseless)
Analgesic Liquid
Antiseptic (mouthwash)
Antacid Gas Tablets
Aspirex Cough Drops
Aspiroids (cold capsules)
Asthmatic Powder
Baby Cough Syrup
Baby Laxative
Beef, Wine and Iron Tonic
Beeveron Tablets; Beeveron Tonic
Bisma-Rex (antacid powder)
Blackberry and Ginger Extracts with
    Carminatives
Branchiol Soothing Tablets
Bunion Pads, Zinc Oxide
Carbolated Witch Hazel Ointment
Carbolic Salve
Castor Oil Compound (aromatic)
Cathartic Pills
Charcoal Tablets
Cherrosote
Cherry Bark Flavored Cough Syrup
Chilblain Lotion
Children's Cough Syrup
Cod Liver Oil Emulsion
Cold Sore Lotion
Compound Mustard-Camphor-Menthol
    Ointment
Corn Pads, Zinc Oxide
Corn Solvent
Denture Adhesive Powder
Denturex (Dental Plate Cleaner)
Deodorant (liquid, cream, or pads)

Diuretic Compound: Diuretic Pills
Emollient Salve
Earache Relief (for pain relief)
Eyelo (eyewash); Eye Drops
Foot Balm; Foot Bath Tablets
Fungi-Rex (for athlete's foot)
Gastric Tablets
GE-7 Effervescent Carbonates
    Compound
Gypsy Cream
Headache Tablets
Hot Carminative Drops
Hygienic Powder
Insect Repellent Cream
Iodized Salve
Iron, Liver and Bone Marrow Com-
    pound
Iron Tonic with Cascara Stomachies
    and Carminatives
Ivy-Chek
Ko-Ko-Kas-Kets
Larkspur Lotion
Lavo-Derma Lotion
Laxative Cold Tablets
Laxative and Diuretic Tea Herbs
Laxative Salt
Malarial Chill Breaker
Maltoleum
Meloids
Melo-Malt Tonic with Cod Liver Oil
Melo-Rex Cough Syrup
Menthol Inhaler
Milk of Magnesia
Milk of Magnesia Tablets
Mi31 Antiseptic Solution
Nasal Jelly with Ephedrine
Nasal Spray with Ephedrine
Nerve Tonic
Neuralgic Tablets

Nucillium
Orderlies
Penetrating Liniment
Pep-Tabs
Peptona
Pile Ointment
Poison Ivy Lotion; Poison Oak Cream
Quick-Acting Liniment
Regs (chocolate-flavored laxative)
Rex-Eme
Rexiltana
Rex-Mentho (chest rub)
Rex-Oleum with Phenolphthalein
Rex-Optex
Rex-Rub
Rex-Salvine
Rex-Seltzer
Rikerdymons
Rubbing Oil
Salicylate Compound
Salicylate Compound Tablets

Salva-Derma Ointment
Sani-Ped Foot Products
Sarsaparilla Flavored Compound with
    Iodide of Potash
Sedets
Seidlitz Powders
Skeeter Skoot
Slippery Elm Lozenges
Sparkling Salts
Spring Tabs
Surgical Powder
Syrup of Figs with Senna
Syrup of Hypophosphites Compound
Throat Lozenges
Toothache Drops
Toothache Wax
Vapure
Vegetable Compound
Vineland Tonic
White Liniment
White Pine, Tar and Wild Cherry

How many of the 1943 list survived the intervening thirty years (since 1913)? Here's the list of products in the line in 1913 and still there thirty years later:

Baby Cough Syrup
Beef, Wine and Iron Tonic
Carbolic Salve
Charcoal Tablets
Cherry Bark Flavored Cough Syrup
Cod Liver Oil Emulsion
Cold Tablets
Corn Solvent
Foot Powder
Pile Treatment
Sarsaparilla Tonic
Vegetable Compound

After the war, product development clearly showed a boost. The following list includes products added to the line in a scant six years since 1943 *(Rexall Almanac):*

Aspirin
Bismo-Rex Mates (tablets)*
Eudicalma Cream or Lotion
Gypsy Cream Ointment*
Iso-Pledrin
Itch Ointment
Klenzo Antiseptic
Laxative Cold Capsules*
Medicated Plasters
Mi31 Throat Tablets*
Milnol
Monacet Compound Tablets
Pabizol
Panovite (multiple vitamins)
Plenamins (multiple vitamins)
Polycaps (children's vitamins)
Prickly Heat Powder
Pro-Cap Adhesive Plasters
Quick Rub
Rexpirin
Rextonia

Finally, Rexall dropped a number of products between 1943 and 1949, including the following *(Rexall Almanac):*

Earache Relief
Iron Tonic Cascara Stomachies and Carminatives
Laxative and Diuretic Tea Herbs
Nerve Tonic
Nucillium
Pep-Tabs
Slippery Elm Lozenges

During this period Rexall worked hard to establish a reputation for quality products. In the 1943 *Rexall Almanac,* the company presented this midwar message.

---

* Indicates dosage form change or addition

"All out"
For production of AMERICA'S HEALTH NEEDS

THESE GREAT FACTORIES

Standing behind the 10,000 Rexall Drug Stores, the factories, warehouses and offices of the great United Drug Company stretch from coast to coast.

Every one of them is now patriotically quickening the mass production of pharmaceuticals, medicines and other drug store needs of the American people. These fresh, potent Rexall Products are shipped direct to Rexall Drug Stores eliminating many of the in-between profits that often boost prices. That's one of the many reasons why you save money when you "buy Rexall."

THIS GREAT DEPARTMENT of RESEARCH and CONTROL

To make sure that every Rexall Product is of the highest quality and purity, the United Drug Company Department of Research and Control must test and approve each one in the laboratory— one of the world's outstanding industrial research laboratories. Here a staff of noted scientists and physicians are constantly at work to make Rexall Products as fine, pure and potent as modern science can achieve.

In 1944 the effort continued:

"Full speed ahead"
For Production of AMERICA'S HEALTH NEEDS

"COME WAR, COME PEACE" THE UNITED DRUG COMPANY stands behind the 10,000 Rexall Drug Stores, as it has stood for more than forty years, to supply you and your family with the comfort and health needs that are a part of America's high standard of living.

The United Drug Company's vast factories, warehouses and offices stretch from coast to coast, as do the Rexall Stores themselves.

As this publication goes to press, two of these factories, manufacturers of the Firstaid Products and Rubber Goods that have long been known to Rexall customers for their quality and dependability, have been awarded the Army and Navy E for distinguished war production. Others, as needed, are engaged in war work of various kinds.

Every one of them is now patriotically working full speed ahead in the mass production of pharmaceuticals, medicines and other drug store needs for the American people at home and abroad. These fresh, potent Rexall Products are shipped direct to Rexall Drug Stores, eliminating many of the in-between profits that often boost prices. That's one of the many reasons why you save money when you "buy Rexall" . . . why you always get the best values in town at your Rexall Drug Store, along with prompt efficient service.

UNITED DRUG COMPANY DEPARTMENT OF RESEARCH and CONTROL, in order to make sure that every Rexall Product is of the highest quality and purity, must test and approve each one in the laboratory—one of the world's outstanding industrial research laboratories. Here a staff of noted scientists and physicians are constantly at work to make Rexall Products as fine, pure and potent as modern science can achieve.

Own Brands and Trailers

Louis Liggett founded United Drug on the concept known today as "store brands," sometimes called private labels. Rexall products were available only to Rexall druggists and to the public only from Rexall druggists. And with only one Rexall druggist in town, there was no competition for the sale of Rexall products. The competition could not engage in price-cutting because they didn't have the products.

The concept initiated and expanded by United Drug relied first and foremost on the quality of the products to which Rexall druggists had exclusive rights. Belief in that quality had to be developed among the druggists and, ultimately, their customers. That was the job of promotion (see Chapter 7) and depended naturally on the ability of the product to live up to promotional claims.

Liggett referred regularly in his Dear Pardner letters and other communications to *own goods,* a wonderful term suggesting personal ownership of Rexall products and reminding the druggists of the value of and need for promoting their own line of products. Liggett also frequently used the term *trailers*. By this he meant products other than the main product being promoted or ones that were not advertised at all. He continued to remind his Pardners not to forget them.

Postwar Product Expansion

By 1950, as reported in that year's annual report, Rexall controlled nine manufacturing facilities:

- St. Louis, Missouri: The home of some 2,400 pharmaceutical and medicine products
- Boston, Massachussets: Cara-Nome cosmetics and Sugar-Free Tooth Paste
- New Haven, Conneticut: Seamless Rubber Company and some first aid products
- Valley Park, Missouri: Most of Rexall's first aid and hospital supplies
- Highland, New York: Chocolate syrup, grape juice, and fountain syrups
- Albany, New York: Stationery and school supplies
- Mansfield, Massachusetts: Rexall candy products
- Williamsport, Pennsylvania: Hosiery products
- Los Angeles, California: Riker Laboratories and prescription products

In 1977, shortly before Rexall would pull the plug on their thousands of franchisees, the *Rexall Drug Company Illustrated Catalog* listed the following for sale:

- Sixteen cough and cold products
- Seven antacids, including Bisma-Rex, a big seller
- Seven systemic analgesics
- A variety of laxatives, sleep aids, diet aids, hemorrhoid remedies, athlete's foot treatments, topical antibiotics, and topical liniments

The vitamin offerings had expanded dramatically (presaging the acquisition by Sundown) to include some sixty individual products, most in more than one strength. Super Plenamins, a major product, received special attention in the catalog. The catalog also offered generic prescription medications, ranging from ampicillin to terpin hydrate and codeine sulfate elixir. In addition (and the irony is almost overwhelming), the catalog offered for sale made-to-order Rexall drugstore signs for shop exteriors. Only a short time later those signs would be coming down.

PRESCRIPTIONS

So far the word *prescription* has only just appeared in a book about the drug business! Of course, in the early days Rexall had no prescription drug products per se (although Riker Laboratories would later offer them). Rexall was aware, however, that prescriptions *were* a product of their druggists' customers. With this in mind, Rexall provided druggists with suggested advertising copy for use in promoting prescription business. Here, verbatim, is the text of a suggested advertisement from 1913:

PARENTS:
Where Are You Going to Get That Prescription Filled?

This is an important question—just as important as your selection of the doctor who writes the prescription.

The slightest departure from the details laid down in that prescription may make it entirely valueless—may mean a delay in the intended relief, resulting in the ailment becoming much more serious and more difficult to relieve.

The welfare of the patient—often even life—depends upon getting your prescription filled exactly as the doctor orders. Economy also demands that there be no shortcoming in the filling of the prescription, for it is usually worthless if not filled right.

When you bring your prescription to us you are absolutely protected. You get what the doctor orders, exactly as he orders it—every specified ingredient in exactly the right proportion, and absolute purity and standard strength.

Your prescription is safe when you bring it here. It is intelligently and honestly filled.

> There is another way in which you best serve economy when you bring your prescription here, *because our prescription prices are lowest, quality considered.*

The Rexall Stores Are America's Greatest Drug Stores.

The people at United were, of course, well aware that a prescription customer represented an opportunity to sell one or more Rexall products, so they found other ways to help their franchisees expand prescription opportunities. For example, the January 1913 issue of *Rexall Ad-Vantages* printed tips from four practicing pharmacists on how they improved their prescription products. Some of those are quite curious today, but one can easily sense the sincerity of these early pharmacists, even though a couple of commercials (for typewriters and labels) did slip in.

C. C. Baer gave some "Prescription Pointers":

> My bottles all carry my name and address on the back, while each cork bears a blue and white sticker on the top.
> Every liquid prescription is filtered, unless it carries some insoluble substances such as the Bismuth Salts. For this purpose I use the bulb stem glass funnel with a small piece of cotton which permits very rapid filtration and does not delay your customer unnecessarily.
> *My labels are all type-written on a Blickensderfer with druggists' attachment.* These little precautions tend to increase the physician's confidence, and the neat appearance increases the patient's faith in the medicine. . . .
> Of course, all Nitrate of Silver solutions *are dispensed in dark bottles, just as all mercurial ointments are handled with a rubber spatula and put out in glass jars.* Powders are evenly folded in waxed papers. Prescriptions are wrapped in white paper and sealed with wax.

William Brennan told of "Getting Rx trade":

> In building a prescription business you must make your strongest appeal to the doctors. . . .
> We make it a point to have the latest drugs in stock, and to keep our prescription men thoroughly posted on doses and prices so that they can answer questions without having to look for information. The doctor is usually in a hurry and does not like

to wait, even for information. We also distribute to the physician circulars on all new drugs and preparations. . . .

We always give a new bottle or box when refilling prescriptions, and we use typewritten labels, thus insuring people against mistakes in reading directions. If a customer does not like to wait, or if it is inconvenient for him to call again, we instruct our clerk to offer to send the prescription without extra charge.

At every opportunity we call the customer's attention to the checking label on the back of our prescription boxes and bottles, emphasizing the fact that there is no danger of mistakes in our store.

Another essential in gaining public confidence is to have always in stock articles that other stores do not carry.

We have made many steady customers just because we happened to have an article in stock which could not be secured elsewhere.

I consider it important to locate the prescription room where people can see the clerks at their work. It creates a favorable impression when customers learn that you have men who devote their whole time to putting up prescriptions.

C. A. Potterfield offered "Prescription Helps":

Use an imported, embossed parchment paper for prescriptions and boxes with a compartment to hold a good maroon rubber dropper for all eye preparations.

In stopping bottles use a celluloid disk through which the cork protrudes, and which covers the lip of the bottle, keeping it free from dust and dirt. . . .

For boxes to contain pills and powders use the finest. You can get them from the New York Label and Box Company. They cost more, but it pays to use your ammunition on the family trade.

A. E. Kiesling presented "How I Sell Prescriptions":

Use red labels and amber bottles for all external preparations. Dispense eye ointments in glass patch boxes.

Always send a dropper with all eye solutions as well as with other liquids to be taken by drops.

Send a camel hair brush with liquids to be applied by this means. Capsules and pills, twenty-four and over, should be dispensed in screw cap bottles.

Do not attempt to fill a prescription by substitutions, or by guessing. If you cannot obtain the preparation, consult the doctor, or return the prescription.

Double check every prescription, using a small check label.

Eye solutions should be dispensed in glass stoppered [G-S] bottles. This avoids any dust from the cork. One-half ounce and one ounce G-S tinctures bottles may be secured from the Illinois Glass Company. . . .

Use good Pill and Powder boxes, and if you do not possess a typewriter for writing labels, buy one at once even if you have to borrow the money.

Riker Laboratories

Although not a part of the main story being told here, mention should be made of Rexall's venture into the manufacture of prescription medications. Riker was the first postwar diversification by Rexall, with the company's first products being marketed in 1950. Before Riker's offerings at least one prescription product, Eudital, was advertised to physicians as a "non-barbituric hypnotic that induces safe, natural sleep," though the ingredients were not identified. Among the better-known prescription products were these:

Medihaler
Norflex
Norgesic
Durophet and Duromine
Rauwiloid
Deaner
Titralac

Of course, Rexallites did not have exclusive rights to these products. Riker was ultimately sold to the 3M Company.

CONCLUSION

The Rexall product strategy certainly changed toward the end. In 1979 President Howard Vander Linden wrote, in the new internal publication *Rexall Review,* "As time goes on, Rexall will become known more as a manufacturing/marketing company and *less as a drug-store-oriented retailer* [emphasis added]."

Chapter 5

The Genius of Rexall Price

INTRODUCTION

As before, price considerations involve two sets of customers for Rexall—drugstore owners and *their* customers. The reader will remember from Chapter 1 that the genesis of United Drug Company had its origins in price considerations. Price-cutting (and therefore profit cutting) was rampant at the turn of the twentieth century. How to combat it? You can't cut prices on products you can't stock and sell. Liggett saw that exclusive products offered protection and opportunity.

As noted in Chapter 4, Rexall products started as what we today call "store brands." Probably the best-known contemporary store brand is Equate, available only at Wal-Mart. Store brands, such as Equate, offer the customer a product that is more or less identical to a brand-name product at a price that is often as much as 30 percent less. Equate bases its success on the phrase *compare to*. Thus, Equate mouthwash will typically bear the suggestion "Compare to Listerine," which of course would bear a considerably higher shelf price than Equate. A measure of the success of this strategy can be seen in the notice on the Listerine bottle: "This Formula is not sold to any retailer as a store brand."

The Equate model was not how Rexall products began their success. There are important differences. Equate belongs to Wal-Mart. The early Rexall products were "own goods" for thousands of independent druggists. Also, in the early days, the "compare to" strategy was not readily available, as few well-known brands were available for comparisons.

Rexall adopted a policy of developing its own line of products and pricing them fairly. No competition meant no competitive price-cutting—none by non-Rexall drugstores because they did not have the products, and none by other Rexall stores because each town or area had only one Rexall store. The policy of selling direct from the manufacturer, United, to the retailer also meant higher profit margins—40 percent—for the retailer because no compensation needed to be made to a middleman/wholesaler. (This would change in later years.)

THE REXALL ONE-CENT SALE

What follows is a partial transcript of *The Jack Benny Program* of February 21, 1954. In this episode, Jack and the cast are preparing to travel to New York by train, and the faithful Rochester is helping Benny pack:

ROCHESTER: "I've got to go to that drug store and get a few things."
BENNY: "What are you going to get?"
ROCHESTER: "Some toothpaste, vitamin tablets, and shampoo."
BENNY: "Rochester, isn't that a Rexall drug store?"
ROCHESTER: "Yes, sir."
BENNY: "Well, they're having a One-Cent Sale. Here's three cents . . . get me the same."

The listening public knew exactly what Jack Benny was talking about. The Rexall One-Cent Sale was so much a part of Americana that it was not even necessary to mention it by name. (Benny also mentioned Owl Drug, owned by United, frequently.) Under the price rubric, the One-Cent Sale stands supreme, but it is not possible to divorce it from promotion. As there is so much to cover under promotion, we won't even try.

Liggett did not invent the One-Cent Sale, but he did perfect it. According to one account (Rexall ms.), the One-Cent Sale idea was first used by the Gray and Worcester Company of Detroit. They started with a two-for-one sale to promote slow-moving merchandise. To the executives' credit, after the first plan failed, they came up with the one-cent-for-the-second-package idea. "Look what 1¢ will buy" was their message. It worked so well that an account of its success was sent to the editor of *Rexall Ad-Vantages*. Liggett, ever alert, read the article and the rest (pardon the cliché) is history. The 1914 One-Cent

Sale was a terrific success and became "the national merchandising feature of the Rexall store."

So how did it work? The plan was simple. Rexall

1. chose the products to be featured;
2. informed druggists well in advance so that they could prepare an order; and
3. began a semiannual sale with major promotional support such that the customer could purchase one package of a featured product at the regular price and a second for a penny.

By everyone's account—Rexall executives, Rexallites, and the general public—this was a tremendous success and continued to be for decades.

Early on, the One-Cent Sale caught fire with Rexall owners. Consider the comments in some of the letters from *Rexall Ad-Vantages* way back in 1918:

> I am a convert to the One-Cent Sale. For years I have been afraid to try it because of the possible adverse effects on my business afterwards. But instead it stimulated it, and we have had many repeat calls for goods which people bought at sale prices and found excellent. (F. G. Hoffman in Wheatland, Wyoming, population 800)

Mr. Hoffman had legitimate cause for concerns. I spoke with more than one Rexallite who remembered seeing some customers only twice a year—at One-Cent Sale time. In spite of this, most Rexall druggists were happy with the One-Cent Sale, as the following notes, again from the March 1918 *Rexall Ad-Vantages,* and statements by Rexall Retirees in Chapter 3 indicate.

> The One-Cent Sale, properly conducted, cannot fail. If we can do this (sell 1,000 pounds of coffee, 50 hot water bottles, etc.) in a little Nebraska town of 459 population, what should the big fellows do? (C. A. Chandler of Merna, Nebraska)

From another Nebraskan:

> Our fourth One-Cent Sale was a big success as the following figures prove:

First sale covering three days	$367.76
Second sale covering three days	$421.19
Third sale covering three days	$409.74
Fourth sale covering three days	$1,192.28

I would call that some increase! But the fact I wish to empha-size is that we Rexallites are too d— skeptical, we are afraid to buy enough goods for a One-Cent Sale. Believe me, I thought I was getting my feet wet on this last sale, but I have found out I did not even touch water. (Edward Wanek, Nebraska)

What follows next requires an understanding of telephone operations early in the twentieth century. From the same *Ad-Vantages:*

Try this plan. At the Iowa meeting a Rexallite stated that he asked operators of the local telephone switch-board to call up rural subscribers giving the dates of his One-Cent Sale. The girls were glad to do this for the promised reward of a box of candy.

Wonder what Ma Bell would think?!

The One-Cent Sale continued for decades. Merwin *(RFA)* called it "one of the most continuously successful merchandising devices in the century"—and surely it was, at least in the drug business. The sale was the recipient of major promotional support in print and broadcast media. The "Talking Penny" provides an excellent example. What follows are excerpts from 1937 radio broadcasts of the *Rexall Magic Hour.* The show was a potpourri of music, humor (usually rather bad), and, most important, commercials for Rexall. The "Talking Penny" (money talks) was one of the players, not simply a commercial an-nouncer. Incorporating the sponsor directly into the program format was a technique later used to great advantage on *The Phil Harris/ Alice Faye Show* which is discussed in detail in Chapter 6. (Older readers will remember that Fibber McGee and Molly found ways to poke fun at their sponsor during the program but still get their com-mercial message across. Harlow Wilcox, who was spokesman for Johnson's wax and the program—Fibber called him "Waxy"—also worked on Rexall shows.) So let's hear "Talking Penny" talk:

PENNY: Hello folks. Yes, I'm the Talking Penny, and am I important in the Rexall drug store? As important as Don Voorhees [the band leader] to the music. [The Talking Penny introduced the acts between commercials, but her real job was clear. As she prepared to introduce another act the "real" announcer stopped her.]

ANNOUNCER: We can't afford another star.

PENNY: Isn't this a Rexall program?

ANNOUNCER: Yes.

PENNY: At Rexall you get two for the price of one, plus one cent. [Not exactly a knee-slapper, but it got the point across reasonably painlessly. She continues on the heels of a song lyric ending with the words *summer night*.]

PENNY: Folks, you don't have to wait for a summer night to find your magic hour. Visit your Rexall store now. [At which point she introduces the "Rexall Man."]

REXALL MAN: Drugdom's biggest event. For four days from Tuesday until Saturday of this week 10,000 Rexall druggists conduct their annual One-Cent Sale. During this sale both the manufacturer and the retailer sacrifice profits (!)* to make friends for Rexall. Listen to these values:
Pure Test Aspirin—quick relief from ordinary pain and headache, 100 tablets in a bottle, forty-nine cents.

PENNY: Add one cent, get 200 tablets for fifty cents.

REXALL MAN: Rexall's Mi31 solution—the finest antiseptic mouthwash made, pint bottle forty-nine cents.

PENNY: Add just one cent. Get two pints for fifty cents.

The broadcast continues with Penny helping the listeners with their math, then "Oh, Mr. Rexall Man, tell them about the Magic Hour." The announcer then describes a special deal on soap, one to a customer, "while supplies last," at opening time on Wednesday.

As the next program opens, the resident tenor sings: "Money talks, tells a merry tale. Money talks, at the One-Cent Sale" and then the spiel begins:

---

* Even on One-Cent Sale merchandise the Rexall druggist made a satisfactory profit. A 1917 One-Cent Sale order blank offers Blackberry Cordial at $9.75 per 100. At a selling price to customers of two for twenty-six cents, the druggist realized a profit of $3.25, or about 25 percent.

ANNOUNCER [Mr. Rexall Man]: Money talks. Just listen to the little coin Rexall has made famous from coast to coast.

PENNY: Friends, Americans and Countrymen, lend me your ears. To hear me talk my loudest, take me with you to a Rexall Drug Store.

Following a musical number or two, Penny continues her conversation with the announcer, reminding him *again* that they can afford another number because it's a Rexall show: "Buy one, get another one for a penny." Then back to the Rexall Man for another special message or special offer—among the products was "Pure Test Cod Liver Oil, used by the Dionne quintuplets, just forty-nine cents." Perky Penny of course reminds the audience about the one cent. A list of a half dozen specials follows the same byplay and finally a note to ask the Rexall druggist for a free coupon "worth forty-nine cents."

ANNOUNCER: This has been a presentation of 10,000 high quality drug stores.

On day three of the sale, Penny chirps in again with the same byplay about being able to afford another musical number because "it's a Rexall show"—a rather effective way of getting the commercial message across. This is followed by the same Rexall Man message—the manufacturer and the retailer are giving up profits—comes a list of additional specials. Penny describes the sale as a way to "save with safety."

Now who could resist a talking penny? Nobody. During the One-Cent Sale crowds of people would buy products. Indeed, in today's environment, the kinds of crowds reported for these sales would pose a serious security problem. Extra clerks would be needed to keep merchandise from leaving the store without even the benefit of the penny.

Another clever ploy was the use of preprinted shopping lists, complete with prices, of goods available during the One-Cent Sale. They were distributed well in advance of the sale to allow a "home inventory" before the fact. Customers simply handed their lists to a clerk and their shopping was painlessly completed. (I can still see in my mind's eye as a youngster a copy of such a list taped to my aunt's refrigerator.)

Another pricing-related item was the ability of druggists to "stock up" for the sale at special low prices. Many of them learned to over-buy, leaving goods with a higher margin for later. In addition to the big sale were frequent specials on product such as Plenamins.

Without question, the One-Cent Sale was the most successful and popular retail event of the twentieth century. More than one Rexallite reported selling more merchandise in those four days than in any one month. Still, the sales did have problems. In 1950 the Federal Trade Commission ordered Rexall to stop misrepresenting prices in con-nection with these sales. They charged that the "regular" prices quoted in Rexall ads were sometimes higher than those charged by other franchisers. Rexall countered that they had already changed their ads and informed the public in a notice in *The Saturday Evening Post.* The matter was dropped.

The genius of the One-Cent Sale will go down in history and re-mains in the minds of many Americans. It even resulted in a stage play (see this chapter's appendix; *Rexall Ad-Vantages,* March 1918). The reader is urged also to read the introductory material of this "play," which was actually performed by United Drug Company em-ployees in January 1918.

This play would never win a Tony, but what it says about the Rexall family should be apparent. These people cared about the company and about one another. What harmony must have prevailed to inspire these busy executives to compose and then perform in their own play? To what purpose? The answer: To share ideas and especially enthusi-asm for the company mission. A cast member, James DeMoville, was one of the original forty stockholders.

CONCLUSION

The One-Cent Sale was an overwhelmingly successful bit of pric-ing strategy. *Everyone* liked it—the public, the Rexall druggists, and Rexall.

APPENDIX

The Awakening of a Rex Allite
A Play in Three Acts

A Riproarious Triumph!
Modern Business Comedy Presented
by United Drug Company Players
An Outline of the Well-Knit Plot—Clever Character
Portrayal by Unsuspected Stars—Potpourri of Business
Doctrine, Worldly Wisdom and Airy Persiflage

First, resembling the Chorus of a Greek tragedy in point of first appearance, but in no other way, comes Charles E. Murnan as preface to the prologue. He wears a business suit about which there is nothing unusual until, putting his hands carelessly into his pockets, he reveals a waistcoat of flaming, maddening crimson, which stirs in everybody but the wearer a homicidal impulse. In a voice more mellowly reminiscent than usual of Ole Virginny, Mr. Murnan congratulates the house on being "all lit up," gives assurance that Boston is the first large city to witness a performance, heretofore given only "in New York and other small villages," and promises that the cast will be found composed "not of plaster of paris," but of real human ability from the United Drug Company.

For the comfort of possible prudes in the audience, he states that the show is absolutely clean, "all the actors having taken a bath in the afternoon." And, he adds, the performance has for its purpose nothing remotely approaching advertising. He says this deliberately, with convincing sincerity, disappearing, then, between the curtains and bringing into view of the audience a huge Jonteel poster attached to the back of his coat. Thus two birds leave the stage, where, seemingly, but one entered.

Prologue. A Dusty Store and a Musty Rexallite

The curtain rises on the main street of a tank town, revealing the exterior of an antediluvian Rexall Store. Rex Allite (Tommy Breen), wearing baggy, mail-order clothes, skew-gee bone glasses and the fatuous smile of arrested development, stands in the doorway, bidding good-bye to A. Real Comer (Royal C. Brown). Comer wears a snappy business suit, carries a suitcase, and is leaving the Rexall Store to make his fortune. He reminds Rex Allite of how he (Comer) has tried to modernize the store, for which he predicts final failure. To

THE AWAKENING OF REX ALLITE
A Business Drama of Modern Merchandising
CAST OF CHARACTERS
In Order of Appearance

KLENZO JONTEE. . . . . C. E. MURNAN
The Business Manager

REX ALLITE . . . . TOMMY BREEN
Who Holds His Pennies So Close to His Eyes He Can't
See a Collar

A REAL COMER . . . . ROYAL C. BROWN
Allite's Clerk, Who Hungers for Progress

A. GREENBACK . . . . C. A. LEAVITT
Who Finally Sells Rex a Cash Register

S. OME QUERIES . . . . E. W. HAWKINS
Who Wants to Know

FULLER PEP . . . . J. L. DEMOVILLE
Who Makes Three Sales Grow Where Before Was Only One

A. PARTICULAR CUSS. . . . . H. J. PURPLE
Who Knows What He Wants

S. LOW MOVER. . . . . H. L. HARDING
Another of Allite's Clerks, Slow at First, but Speedy at Last

P. RESSING. . . . . H. L. SIMPSON
A Drug Jobber Who Insists That "Terms Is Terms—
No Excuses Accepted"

ALL SMILES . . . . HARRY W. TAYLOR
Some Candy Salesman

CON SERVATIVE . . . . J. C. McCORMICK
A Typical Banker

LOTTA SALES . . . . MRS. WALTER STAPLES
Who Makes Penny Sales Grow into Dollars

MISS PURCHASE . . . . MISS MIRIAM D. K. BREEN
A Tractable Customer

Postman and Customers from the Liggett Staff

SILENT ACTORS IN THE DRAMA, unseen by the audience, but contributing nonetheless to the success of the performance: C. A. Merrill, whose good judgment and quick action facilitated the display changes of The Rexall Store; L. S. Crone, who acted as stage manager and prompted the actors.

which Rex Allite replies: "Those fairy tales in business magazines are written by dreamers. I inherited this business from my father. He made a living, and I'm making a living, ain't I?"

Exit Comer, and enter a postman, from whom Rex Allite grouchily grabs his copy of AD-VANTAGES, which he yanks from its wrapper, tears in two, and slams to the sidewalk, muttering, "Huh! Another copy of that circus magazine." *Curtain.*

Act I, Scene 1. Help Arrives

Two years have elapsed. The setting of the first act is that of the prologue. Enter Fuller Pep (Jim DeMoville) and A. Greenback (C. A. Leavitt), the former representing United Drug Company, the latter a cash register manufacturer. A brief colloquy ensues; then exit Greenback as Fuller Pep enters the Rexall Store. *Curtain.*

Act I, Scene 2. A Punk Reception

The curtain rises on the dusty shelves, deadwood stock and dilapidated showcases of "The Central Pharmacy," prototype of many a real drug store. Rex Allite is revealed sprawled at his desk, reading a country newspaper, and giving a lifelike imitation of a dose of morphine. To Fuller Pep's self-introduction he pays no heed. Neither does he hear an impatient customer, who raps a nickel on the cigar case, and leaves disgusted. Idling back of the counter is the mentally anemic, spineless clerk, S. Low Mover (H. L. Harding), exhausted by the strain of watching the clock.

Then follows another customer, S. Ome Queries (E. W. Hawkins) who asks for a feeding tube. Of course the clerk cannot find it, and Rex Allite will not even look for it. At last, accidentally, its location is discovered, and S. Low Mover, throwing it on the counter and poking his thumbs into the armholes of his vest, stares at the customer, who marches out, as he would in real life, succinctly expressing his views in the words "Some service!!!"

Meanwhile Fuller Pep directs a drum-fire of pertinent questions at Rex Allite, who shamelessly admits that he does not know the value of his own merchandise stock, that he never stopped to figure percentages, and that it doesn't matter anyway, since what he owns is *all* his. Fuller Pep's explanation of the importance of inventory in connection with fire insurance, and of the impossibility of figuring profits without knowing operating expense, serves only to antagonize Rex Allite, in whose dull lexicon of age there is no such word as Success.

But Rex Allite is galvanized into something resembling activity, when his landlord telephones a demand for rent, which is ten days overdue. The landlord's brusqueness ruffles the druggist, and from mere rudeness his manner to Fuller Pep becomes insulting. Enter then P. Ressing (H. L. Simpson), a drug jobber, who storms up to the desk, his arms waving, his face red (Simpson can make even his circulatory system act), and delivers his ultimatum: "Got your order, Allite, in this morning's mail, but 'nothing doing' until you pay your past due account."

Rex Allite tries to placate P. Ressing and hide his confusion from Fuller Pep. The jobber's man, however, is adamant. The debtor has been "getting slower and slower in paying bills for the past two years; and, emphasizing by a clenched fist his entire lack of confidence in Rex Allite's ability to make good, he shouts, "Terms is terms! No excuses accepted!" and departs like a thunderstorm that means to come back again.

Seeing the futility of further argument, Fuller Pep also leaves, as Rex Allite grabs the telephone.

He calls the First National Bank and asks for $1,000 on his sixty days' note. The audience hears only half the conversation, but the drift is clear. The bank will lend no money to a man who has neither collateral nor business system. Rex Allite is stunned.

Enter then a radiant self-confident sunbeam in the person of All Smiles (Harry W. Taylor), programmed as "Some Candy Salesman," which he is, off stage and on. All Smiles tries to talk candy profits from Rex Allite's viewpoint.

Exasperated, Rex Allite, with childish petulance, whines, "What I need right now is *money,* not candy." Then he tells how Fuller Pep tried to teach him his business. If he expects commiseration from All Smiles, he hears instead, "You need new life in this store. My advice is to get Fuller Pep back." Exit All Smiles.

Torn by conflicting emotions, Rex Allite fidgets in his chair, then impulsed by the kindly Fates, he telephones Fuller Pep to "come back."

And back he comes after a brief interval, an interval sufficient, however, for S. Low Mover to lose a few more customers. Again Fuller Pep explains the Sales Promotion Plan, and this time the druggist listens. It is the supper hour and S. Low Mover, making his first quick move, heads for the door. He is halted by Fuller Pep, and before he knows what has happened, his hat and coat are off, and under Fuller Pep's direction he is blowing dust from the ancient stock while Fuller Pep takes inventory. The latter, with a kindly pat on the shoulder, sends poor old Rex Allite home to rest, promising to meet him in the morning for a conference with his banker and the jobber. *Curtain.*

Act II, Scene 1. The New Life Begins to Work

The curtain rises on the interior of the Central Pharmacy. S. Low Mover, now spick and span in a white shirt, an audible suit, and with a flower in his buttonhole, is dusting displays. He is actually moving fast. As he works he whistles cheerfully; he is alert, intelligent, ambitious. Enter Rex Allite, who stands amazed at the transfiguration of his employee. The latter proceeds to sing the praises of Fuller Pep, whom he describes as "some pumpkins," and to whom he gives credit for the fact that he himself feels "all made over."

Enter now Fuller Pep, his name justified by his quick step, firm handclasp and buoyant optimism. He announces himself ready for the conference, and as he states the fact, enter P. Ressing, the drug jobber, and Con Servative (J. C. McCormick), a typical banker. Con Servative is immaculately dressed, tall, dignified, courteous, but obviously not sentimental. His speech is incisive, he deals definitely with facts and figures, and explains affably but unequivocally that his bank, despite their confidence in Mr. Rex Allite, etc., etc., cannot loan money to a business that is not scientifically conducted. Abashed by this refusal and further flabbergasted by the drug jobber's continual reiteration of his confounded "Terms is terms! No excuses accepted," Rex Allite turns for support to Fuller Pep. The latter outlines his proposition, convincing both the banker and the jobber that it will rehabilitate the druggist's business. As a clincher, Fuller Pep adds that his own firm is one of Rex Allite's largest creditors, notwithstanding which, realizing the profit-possibilities of the Central Pharmacy when properly conducted, he is disposed to continue his relations with Rex Allite. Impressed by Fuller Pep's frankness, Con Servative promises to lend the druggist $1,000 on a ninety-day note, Rex Allite agreeing to Fuller Pep's suggestion that half of that amount shall be paid to the jobber and the other half used as working capital in the store.

Rex Allite, his burden of worry lifted, faces the future with a smile. *Curtain.*

Mr. DeMoville's Inter-Act Lecture

During the interval between the second and third acts, Manager James L. DeMoville of the Sales Promotion Department gave a stereopticon lecture, illustrating the value of his Service in the Rexall Stores.

Act III, Scene 1. A Day of Prosperity

In the last act the curtain rises on the interior of the Central Pharmacy. Two weeks have elapsed. Only two weeks, but enough for the Sales Promotion Service to get in its work. And what a transformation! The fixtures are bright with varnish, the showcases gleam, the dusty tincture bottles have been replaced by orderly rows of new sight-selling merchandise.

But where is Rex Allite? Can it be that this smooth-shaven, smartly dressed, active, progressive businessman is the same doddering commercial imbecile who tripped on his whiskers in Act II? Yes, it is the very same. He shares his altered demeanor with the erstwhile bookworm victim S. Low Mover, who, having dropped the negative portion of his name, in dropping his negative attitude toward life, is now known—and respected—as Mr. Mover.

Rex Allite holds in his hand an object which, though inanimate, speaks volumes for the modernized store. *It is a Daily Sales Sheet.*

Since the last act, the sales force has been augmented by Miss Lotta Sales (Mrs. Walter Staples) "who makes penny sales grow into dollars." She appeals to women by her insight into their preferences, and, with her quick smile, trim figure, and charming manner, at once safely demure and slightly provocative, is distinctly restful to the masculine eye.

Enter then, to rest his eyes, A. Particular Cuss (H. J. Purple), a customer "who knows what he wants" on the stage, and in real life knows what the public wants in stationery values.

He asks for Rexall Shaving Cream. Mover, stepping briskly, puts his hand unerringly on the right package, and while wrapping it up, gives a talk on Rexall Shaving Lotion, which results in a double sale.

At this juncture re-enter All Smiles, the candy salesman. Rex Allite hails him as a friend, and Smiles, after a characteristic acknowledgment of the beauty of Rex Allite's candy display, outlines a movie-slide plan, wherewith Rex Allite can vastly increase his sales. That worthy, no longer suspicious of things new, promptly orders 500.

It is a busy day for the Central Pharmacy. Enter now Miss Purchase (Miss Miriam D. K. Breen), a charming bit of femininity, who proves to be "a tractable customer." She asks merely for a five-cent rubber nipple, but under the skillful manipulation of Lotta Sales, she is psychologized from one department of the store to another until her purchases include a twenty-five-cent Stork Nurser outfit, a Rexall Comfy Soother, a bottle of Mother Kroh's Teething Syrup, a Kodak with which to take pictures of the baby, two rolls of film, a photograph album and a tube of Old Colony Library Paste.

Oh, the late Professor William James had nothing on Lotta Sales, when it comes to analyzing the human mind! Smilingly she rings the cash register, the audience seeing not the figures "5¢," but $7.85.

Follow now in rapid succession other customers, who are waited on with smiling celerity and profitable proficiency by Lotta Sales and Mr. Mover. The only delay occurs when Rex Allite sends Mr. Mover to the bank with a wad of mazuma, which, by clogging the cash register, had become a deterrent to business.

Again through the throng reappears Fuller Pep accompanied by P. Ressing, the drug jobber, now his real self as he is known off stage, accompanied by Con Servative. The trio shake hands with Rex Allite; there is an interval of mutual congratulation, P. Ressing thanks the druggist for a check recently received, Con Servative looks about the attractive store with obvious approval, and Fuller Pep, proud that his Service has brought order out of chaos, invites his friends to view Rex Allite's window display. Exeunt Fuller Pep, Con Servative, P. Ressing and Rex Allite.

Act III, Scene 2. A Joyful Finale

The curtain rises on the exterior of the Central Pharmacy, revealing a series of wonderfully attractive panel window displays. Con Servative and P. Ressing agree "that the windows certainly are attractive." The drug jobber and Con Servative fully sympathize with Rex Allite when the latter says, "It's certainly remarkable the amount of merchandise that can be sold by Fuller Pep's system."

As his friends depart, Rex Allite is confronted by the postman, from whom he receives once more a copy of AD-VANTAGES. This time he turns its pages carefully, and with a sense of ownership. And to Fuller Pep's parting promise to send Tommy Breen to help him conduct a One-Cent Sale, the new merchant of a new era replies: I'll follow any suggestion you make. *I am wide awake now."* Curtain.

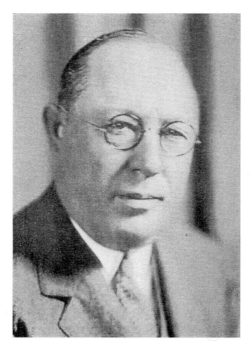
Louis K. Liggett (*Source:* From the author's private collection.)

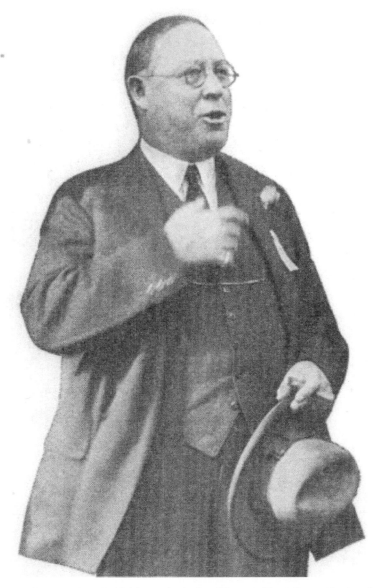

Candid Picture of Louis K. Liggett in Action (*Source:* From the author's private collection.)

REXALL

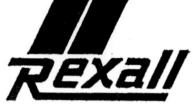

Rexall Logos (*Source:* From the author's private collection.)

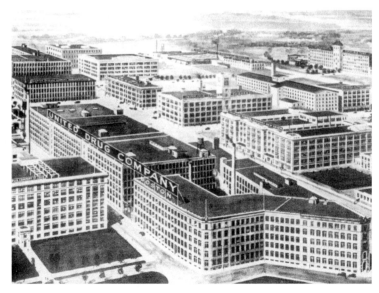

United Drug Headquarters in Boston (*Source:* From the author's private collection.)

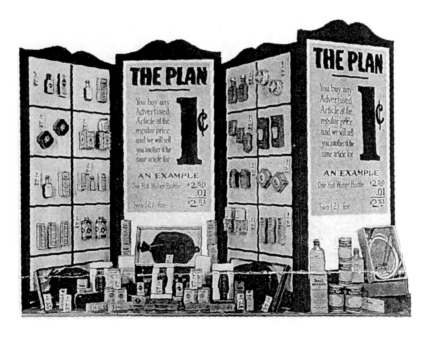

One-Cent Sale Display (*Source:* From the author's private collection.)

One-Cent Sale Order Blank (*Source:* From the author's private collection.)

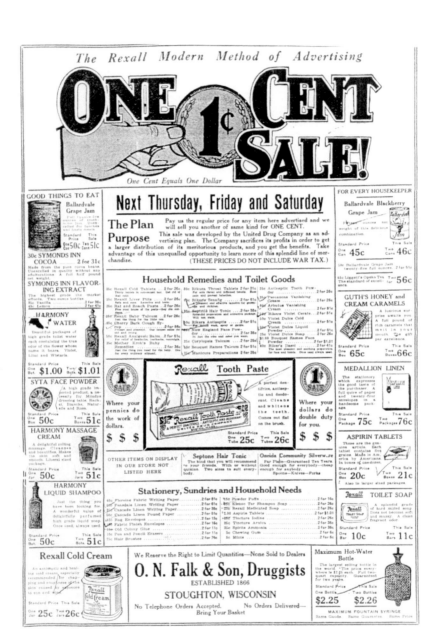

Retail Ad for One-Cent Sale (*Source:* From the author's private collection.)

"THEY'RE OFF"

5000 in the Air at One Time

Look Up, This Isn't April Fool, but Merely an Announcement of The Great

INTERNATIONAL REXALL PIGEON DERBY

At St. Louis Sept. 28--Oct. 1st

Ad for Rexall Pigeon Derby (*Source:* From the author's private collection.)

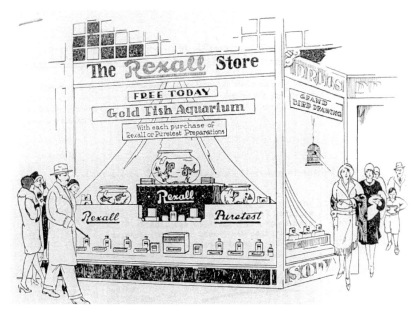

Rexall Goldfish Promotion (*Source:* From the author's private collection.)

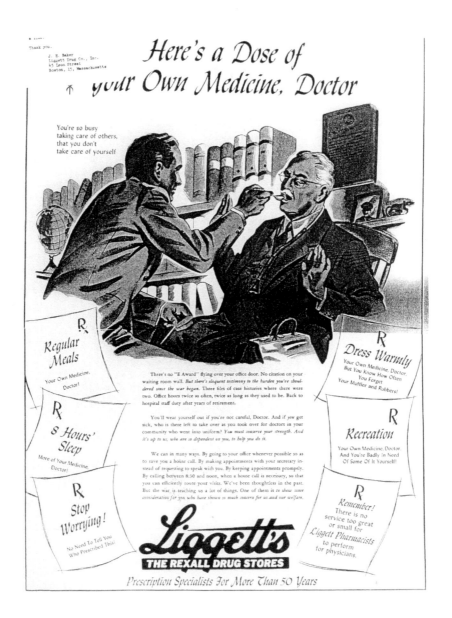

Ad Directed to Physicians (*Source:* From the author's private collection.)

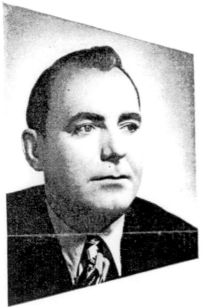

for your summer listening pleasure
we again proudly present...

The Rexall Theatre

starring
PAT O'BRIEN
and Virginia Bruce

You enjoyed it last summer. Now, hear it

again — the exciting drama of the corner drug

store, Crossroads of America.

Spend a pleasant half hour with Pat O'Brien

in the role of the pharmacist, and his friends

and neighbors. It's your story...about

your people...in

Yourtown, U. S. A.

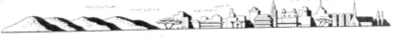

NBC

SUNDAY NIGHTS — COAST TO COAST

*   *   *

Promotion for the *Dan Carson Show (Source:* From the author's private collection.)

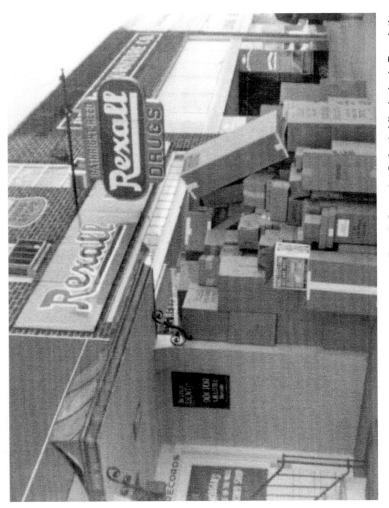

Merchandise for One-Cent Sale Arrives at a Rexall Store in Oxford, Mississippi, Population About 7,000 at the Time (*Source:* Photo courtesy of Aston Holley.)

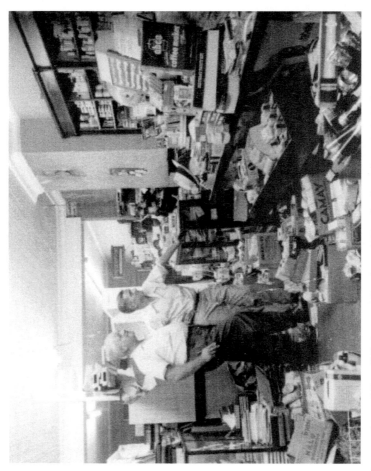

Pharmacist and Rexall Salesman Study and Plan for One-Cent Sale in Oxford, Mississippi (*Source:* Photo courtesy of Aston Holley.)

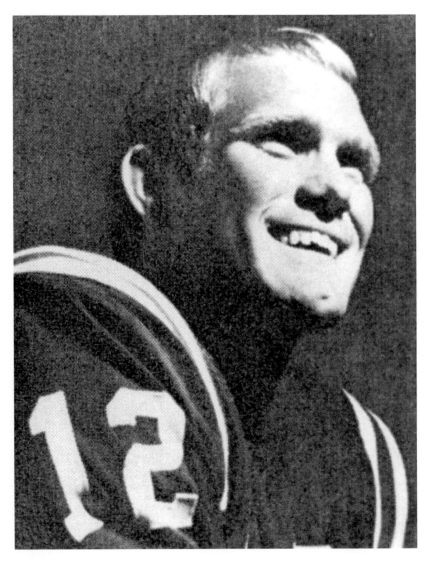

Terry Bradshaw, Number One NFL Draft Choice, 1970, Endorses Super Plenamins
(*Source:* From the author's private collection.)

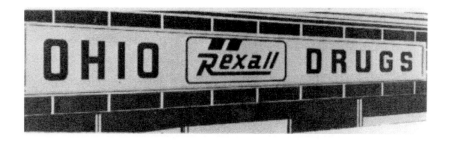

Rexall Catalog Ad Offering Rexall Signs (*Source:* From the author's private collection.)

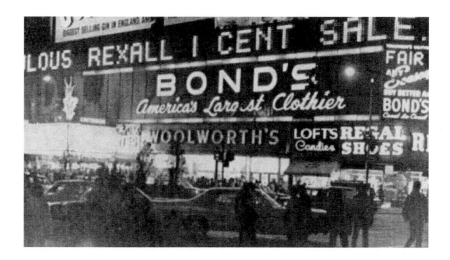

One-Cent Sale Advertised in Times Square (*Source:* From the author's private collection.)

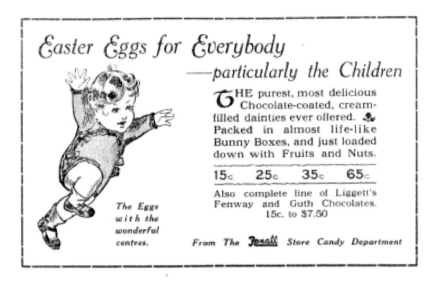

Easter Eggs for Everybody

—particularly the Children

THE purest, most delicious Chocolate-coated, cream-filled dainties ever offered. Packed in almost life-like Bunny Boxes, and just loaded down with Fruits and Nuts.

15c   25c   35c   65c

Also complete line of Liggett's Fenway and Guth Chocolates. 15c. to $7.50

The Eggs with the wonderful centres.

From The Rexall *Store Candy Department*

Run this Ad at Easter Time

We'll be glad to furnish the cut and copy FREE as indicated on the Order Blank. The Kiddie appeals to grown-ups, and used in your advertising creates the necessary punch. This Kiddie cut is also on the big window strip, coming to you FREE with each shipment. Tie together your window and newspaper advertising.

Sample Ad Supplied to Stores (*Source:* From the author's private collection.)

A New Profit Maker

A Combination Greeting Card and Special Drug Sundries Case that will Revolutionize Sales for *Rexall* Drug Stores

Briefly This Announcement Means—

You can now get your share of fifty million dollars of greeting card sales, and selling will be a pleasure.

You can get the valuable other trade that comes from greeting card buyers coming to your store.

You can handle all sizes and kinds of cards without confusion or waste of space.

In **three minutes** you can change the card case into a special sales case that will move any "sticker."

UNITED DRUG COMPANY

BOSTON, MASS.

Ad to Stores for Greeting Cards (*Source:* From the author's private collection.)

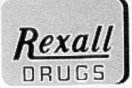

FRANCHISE
AGREEMENT

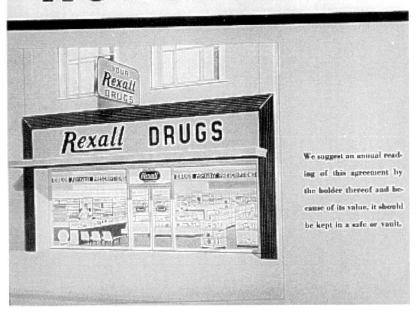

We suggest an annual reading of this agreement by the holder thereof and because of its value, it should be kept in a safe or vault.

Franchise Agreement Booklet Cover (*Source:* From the author's private collection.)

REXALL FRANCHISE AGREEMENT

AGREEMENT made this_____ day of_____, 19____ between **REXALL DRUG COMPANY**, a Delaware corporation, with principal office in Los Angeles, California, (hereinafter called "REXALL") and

_____

the Sole Ownership
a Partnership   (of) (consisting of) _____
a Corporation

_____

_____

_____ (hereinafter called "RETAILER").

WITNESSETH:

It is mutually agreed as follows:

SECTION 1. REXALL hereby appoints RETAILER as a REXALL DEALER and authorizes him to designate his store as a REXALL DRUG STORE. RETAILER may use the words "REXALL DRUGS" in conjunction with his own name in store identification signs, advertising material, letterheads and the like but shall not include the word "REXALL" in the firm, corporate, or tradename under which he does business.

SECTION 2. REXALL hereby grants to RETAILER the right to sell REXALL MERCHANDISE, as hereinafter defined, at retail only, at

No._____ Street, in the City

or Town of _____ State of _____, but not elsewhere.

SECTION 3. REXALL agrees to supply REXALL MERCHANDISE to RETAILER in the regular course of its business and upon the regular terms made by it to other REXALL DEALERS. RETAILER agrees to promptly pay for all such merchandise in accordance with the regular terms made by REXALL. Wherever the words "REXALL MERCHANDISE" are used in this agreement, the same shall be taken to mean that merchandise which REXALL may from time to time offer to its REXALL DEALERS.

SECTION 4. RETAILER agrees to:

(a) Use his best efforts and facilities at all times to establish, maintain and increase the sale of REXALL MERCHANDISE; keep on hand at all times a representative stock of such merchandise sufficient to supply the demand therefor and give such merchandise first preference in display, advertising and sale. He shall always bring such merchandise to the attention of the public and shall always sell the same when called for and when opportunity offers.

(b) Identify his store as a REXALL DRUG STORE by the installation and maintenance in good order and condition of such official orange and blue REXALL signs, REXALL valances, and REXALL decalcomanias as REXALL shall consider adequate for RETAILER'S location.

(c) Support all REXALL national advertising by paying for and using the monthly Sales Promotion Service and purchasing each month REXALL MERCHANDISE sufficient to properly support the event.

(d) Advertise locally and actively promote in his store all REXALL Major Promotions. Major Promotions shall include the Fall and Spring One-Cent Sales and such other sales as REXALL may from time to time so designate.

(e) Share proportionately with other REXALL DEALERS and REXALL in the cost of the REXALL National Cooperative Advertising Program. RETAILER'S share shall not exceed two and one-half per cent (2½%) of his aggregate purchases from REXALL.

SECTION 5. This agreement may be terminated by RETAILER on giving thirty (30) days' written notice to REXALL.

FORM #1000 - REVISED 11/68

Franchise Agreement Opening Page (*Source:* From the author's private collection.)

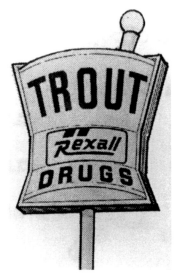

Another Sample Rexall Sign for Sale (*Source:* From the author's private collection.)

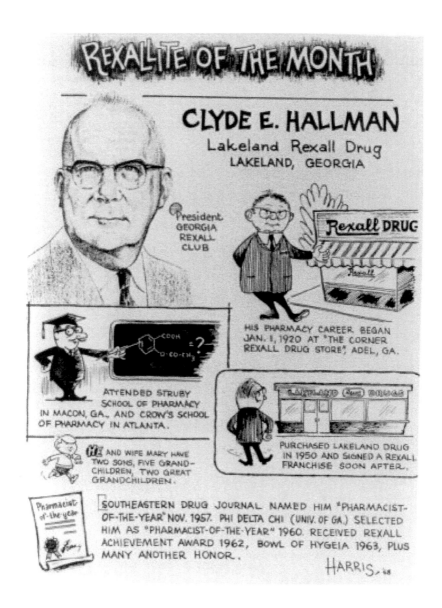

Example of Recognition of Franchises (*Source:* From the author's private collection.)

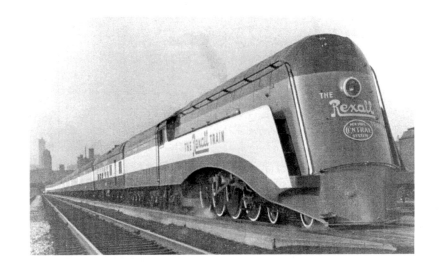

View of the Rexall Train (*Source:* Collection of Harold K. Vollrath.)

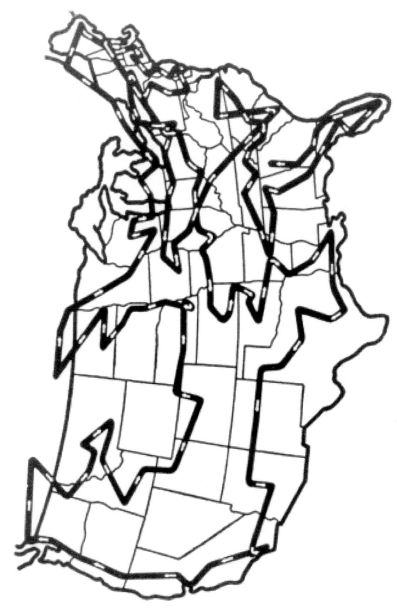

Route of the Rexall Train (*Source: Courtesy of the Terminal Railroad Association of St. Louis.*)

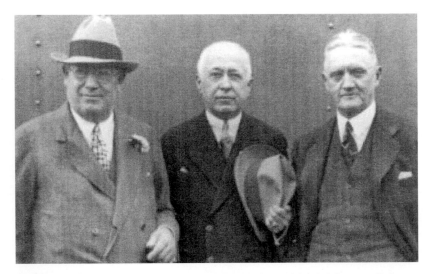

Admit Mr. *S. Y. WHITNEY*

(Good for ONE ADULT)

TO THE EXHIBITS ON THE

REXALL STREAMLINED TRAIN

AT NORTH STATION, BOSTON

Friday, March 27th, 9 A. M. to 4 P. M.
Sunday, March 29th, 10 A. M. to 4 P. M.

PRESENT THIS TICKET AT TRAIN ENTRANCE

Rexallite: To validate this ticket please fill in above and sign.

Rexallite's Name

Town

Ticket to the Train (*Source:* Courtesy of the Terminal Railroad Association of St. Louis.)

(Left to Right) Liggett, Harry Dockum (a Rexall Director), and George Gales at the Train (*Source:* Photo courtesy of the Terminal Railroad Association of St. Louis.)

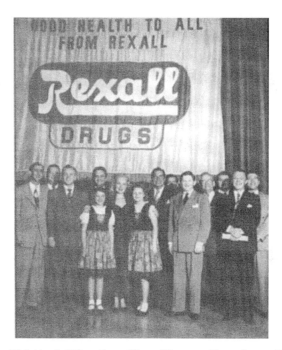

Cast of *The Phil Harris/Alice Faye Show* (*Source:* From the author's private collection.)

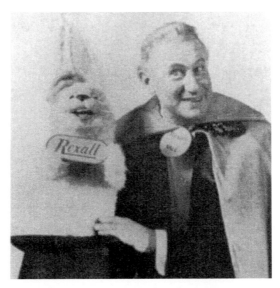

TV Magician "Rexall the Great" (*Source:* From the author's private collection.)

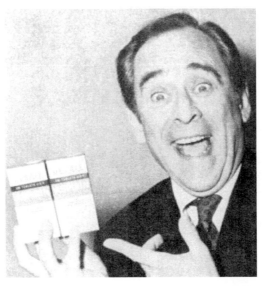

Louis Nye Hawks Rexall on TV (*Source:* From the author's private collection.)

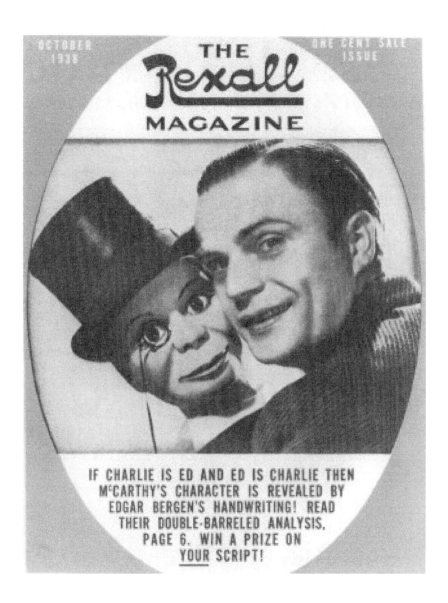

Cover of Consumer-Oriented *Rexall Magazine* (*Source:* From the author's private collection.)

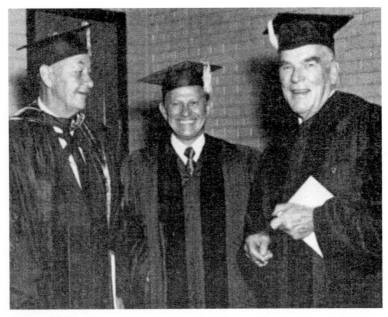

Justin Dart (Right) Receives Honorary Doctor of Laws Degree from University of Southern California (*Source:* From the author's private collection.)

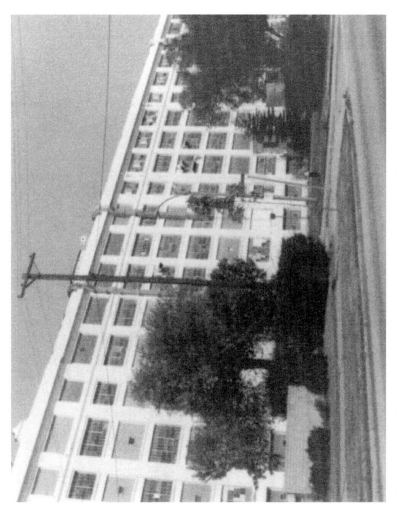

Rest in Peace: Rexall Headquarters in St. Louis in Better Days (*Source:* From the author's private collection.)

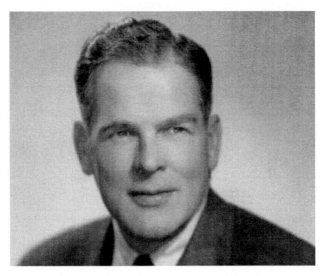

Justin Dart at His Peak (*Source:* From the author's private collection.)

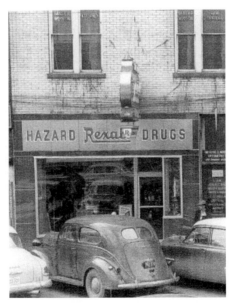

Hazard Rexall Drugs in 1953 When Duncan Had Just Purchased It (*Source:* From the author's private collection.)

Chapter 6

The Genius of Rexall Place

In the academic study and teaching of marketing, the third P—place—usually gets the least attention and seems to be considered to be the least interesting. Place includes the distribution function and is much more interesting than is usually believed. It is especially worth the reader's time.

THE REXALL PLACE CONCEPT

Merwin (*RFA*, p. 17) had this to say about Liggett: "He is a channel opener, a simplifier. He serves. He helps to build the concerns with which he deals. He serves."

Louis Liggett's vision of place was unique for its time. It combined exclusivity (only one franchise in an area) with universal availability to consumers (a Rexall store in every county was Liggett's goal). Added to that was the typical location of Rexall drugstores. They didn't call them corner drugstores for nothing!

This was designed as a win-win situation. United Drug gives the druggists exclusive rights to buy and sell its products. Druggists agree to buy them and put their best efforts into selling them. The more they sell, the more money they make and, of course, the more money United Drug/Rexall makes.

Reading historical accounts and Dear Pardner letters, it is obvious that this was more than just good business for United/Rexall. For many, the company provided a sense of family spirit. The motto "All for One and One for All" was frequently quoted.

PHYSICAL DISTRIBUTION

The place concept just described was important, but other conditions were (and are) the basic nuts and bolts of the physical distribution of the products to the drugstores. Druggists couldn't sell what they didn't have, so timeliness of delivery was essential. Some problems early on involved the state of transportation at the time. In 1917, for example, it was necessary to establish an intercity freight truck service between the Boston headquarters and New York City. Some fifteen trucks were needed for the round-trip which took five days (Rexall ms.). Today, of course, most druggists order electronically for next-day delivery, but that is usually through a wholesaler, not direct from the manufacturer, as was the case with Rexall.

As time and success moved rapidly toward a national network of druggists, a national distribution system became a necessity. This was accomplished over time by the establishment of a series of warehouses to ensure more timely delivery, beginning as early as 1916 with a West Coast Branch warehouse in San Francisco, followed by one in St. Louis and one in Chicago.

Efficient and timely distribution required cooperation of the druggists themselves. A letter (dated April 10, 1917) from H. B. Storm of the One-Cent Sale Department provides a good example:

Dear Rexallite:

We have just received advice from the Chicago Branch, and the same is perhaps true at the St. Louis Branch as well, that a good many of the stockholders wire, write or telephone the Branches for One-Cent Sale merchandise while their One-Cent Sale is going on, for goods that they are running short of, or have run out of entirely.

The Branches cannot under any circumstances take care of these orders. All One-Cent Sale merchandise at this time is especially keyed with the letter "K" and none of this keyed merchandise is carried at the Branches.

Therefore, if you run out of any item during your One-Cent Sale, or if you see that you are not going to have enough of any item to take care of your demand, it will be necessary that you handle it the same as previously instructed—that is, take orders with promise of delivery of the goods after your Sale is over, and then send the list of goods needed to Boston, using the *Over-Sold Order Blank* which is supplied you with your One-Cent Sale invoice, and we will take care of you as promptly as possible, and *bill you at the One-Cent Sale price.*

The above explains that the Chicago Branch and also the St. Louis Branch cannot honor your order under any circumstances, and if they receive your order it means that they will ship you the goods and bill you at the regular price, and not at the One-Cent Sale price. This means that goods ordered from the Branches to be sold on the One-Cent Sale plan would be a loss to you on the majority of items ordered.

CHANNEL RELATIONSHIPS

Contemporary marketing texts treat the way distribution is handled using the term *channel relationships*—meaning the ways conflict and cooperation affect the efficiency and effectiveness of the distribution system from manufacturer to consumer. United/Rexall took channel relationships seriously from the outset and used a variety of media to ensure good relationships.

Letters

Chapter 2 focused on the Dear Pardner letters sent twice monthly from President Liggett himself. They ranged from folksy "We're all in this together"—to serious attention to issues affecting both parties. These were not the only letters sent to Rexall druggists, however.

Over the years Rexallites received hundreds of letters from various executives in the United Drug Company that included tips on merchandising, special offers, notices of new products, and sometimes just encouragement. Although some of what follows might belong in Chapter 7's discussion of promotion, it is included here because it represents efforts by United to help their clients do well. (The reader is referred to the picture section for other examples.)

In a 1925 letter, the manager of toilet goods specialists provided Rexallites with the following sample promotional letter:

Dear Madam:

An opportunity has presented itself which I am sure will be of interest and benefit to you.

We have been successful in securing the services of a scientifically trained Toilet Goods Specialist for one week beginning [date].

If you wish to keep your skin soft, smooth, and fresh, the pores must be cleaned daily from impurities such as dust or an accumulation of natural secretion in the skin, both of which, if allowed to remain, clog the pores and give rise to skin troubles. The complexion fades from neglect and must not be slighted.

Face massage should be performed at home and the treatment is very simple. The Toilet Goods Specialist will teach you the proper method of caring for the complexion as well as the scalp and hair. She will only be able to fill a limited number of engagements, and we want to give you the very first opportunity. All I ask of you is a manifestation of your interest to the extent of giving only thirty minutes of your time for a free facial massage.

If you are interested and will phone us in the next day or two, we will be glad to make a definite engagement.

He didn't stop there, however. He explained in detail what was necessary—a recipe for success:

This is an age of keen competition and I know of no merchandise that is more subject to trade rivalry than the toilet goods line. Therefore, in 1925, let us put forth every effort to keep before the women of your community the toilet items for which you have the exclusive sales privilege.

Efficiency Experts tell us that success or failure in any line of business rests primarily with those who come into direct contact with the buying public. You know that sales depend on public confidence in merchandise and service, and there is no better way to win and hold public confidence and increase the volume of your controlled goods business than by conducting demonstrations of OWN GOODS.

In order to make this demonstration a phenomenal success it is absolutely necessary for you and your salespeople to cooperate to the fullest extent with the Toilet Goods Specialist. If properly managed the demonstrations will be productive of excellent results.

Be sure that you have at least FIFTY APPOINTMENTS for the Specialist for the week.

Also see that the Complete Cara-Nome line is displayed in show-cases, on counters and case tops and in your windows before the arrival of the Specialist.

It costs you over $5.00 per day for the services of the Specialist. Assuredly then, it is to your advantage to make the appointments, since if you keep her busy the results will be most gratifying. The Specialist will work hard to please your customers, and I know that she will make many boosters for your complete toilet goods line.

A brilliant sample letter (date undocumented) to a newborn was provided in another message for the Rexallite. What better way to touch the heart of a new mother?

Dear Baby:

We have just heard of your arrival in this big round world. We are glad you have come and we bid you welcome.

We love babies and we know their little troubles. Some of these nights you will have a "tummy ache," so we are sending you a cute little hot water bottle just big enough to cover the "hurtie" place. When you have a little pain, ask mama to fill your little bottle with hot water, put it on your little "tummy" and it will help a lot. Some day when you are out in your little traveling carriage, ask your mamma to bring you into the Rexall store so we may become acquainted.

When you are big enough to do errands for your mother you will always come here—all the children do—because we treat little folks just as nicely as we do big folks. You will always have a friend in this store. With lots of love and good wishes for your future, we are always,

Yours truly,
W. S. Hufford

P. S. The Hot Water Bottle spoken of by Mr. Hufford is the Petite Face Bottle R. 94. Of course, any other Hot Water Bottle or article could be used, such as, can of talc, castile soap, etc., but he found the Hot Water Bottle more effective.

Equally brilliant was a sample letter to newcomers (women)— a perfect way to be the first welcoming druggist in town:

Dear Madam:

We wish to welcome you to our neighborhood and we trust you will be delighted with our city.

Our store is very centrally located and easily reached from all parts of the town. Our customers know our store gives intelligent and quick service and we hope you will give us a trial to show how well we can take care of your business.

We are sole agents for all the lines of the United Drug Company, including the celebrated Rexall line. We have such confidence in all the goods manufactured by this company that we sell them on absolute guarantee to give satisfaction.

Our prescription department is in the hands of registered pharmacists and we guarantee to fill your prescriptions with the very finest materials obtainable.

Our delivery service is prompt and we will be glad to have your telephone orders at any time. To induce you to give us a call, we will give you free with the first dollar purchase a 25¢ can of Jonteel Talc and we feel sure you will think it the most delightful talcum you have ever tried.

Yours very truly,

THE REXALL STORE

It is my personal opinion that Rexallites were provided with a treasure chest of promotional tips. If all had used them, with judgment and selectivity, I sincerely believe that the "ten thousand" Rexall druggists would have become a retail juggernaut that no one could have ignored.

Other Examples

Rexall did not simply preach but also attempted to receive feedback. In an undated questionnaire, druggists were offered the chance to give their opinions:

Your frank answers to the following questions will improve your SALES PROMOTION SERVICE. Fill out, sign and return to Sales Promotion Dept. Boston.

Do you like the panel arrangement of displays?
Should you have any more panels?
Do you like the tinted backgrounds?
Are the five showcards enough for each display?
Would you suggest any alterations in the selling talks?
Would you suggest any alterations in advertisements?
Is the price ticket arrangement satisfactory?
Do you receive your display material on time?
Are two displays a week sufficient?
Are you using the daily and weekly sales sheets?
Are you using the Suggestion Cards?
Have you any suggestions for the improvement of the Service?

Practical matters were addressed as well. In 1924 the manager of the candy department advised:

Beginning June 1st the Chicago and St. Louis Branches, whenever in their judgement it is necessary to furnish protection from the heat [before the days of refrigerated trucks], will ship candy by express prepaid to you, charging you 50 percent of the express cost only, and that 50 percent will be added to the face of the invoice.

Why pay this?

Well you know that there is about as much candy eaten in the summer as any other time, but when you slow up your efforts naturally the candy public are not as tempted as they are at other times of the year.

There was no limit to the tips provided. The following sample letters were provided to Rexallites to deal with past-due accounts. (If the Rexallites got into financial trouble in this way, they were of little good to Rexall.) The sequence of three sample letters, beautifully composed and dated 1918, are preceded by an explanation.

From United

But you may ask, what am I to do when my collection efforts fail, and I believe the customer cannot pay?

You might well go on and say, "These people are my good friends and neighbors and I am sorry for them. We want their cash business. They are not going to leave town; they will still need drugs, toilet articles, etc.; they can get better goods and service from us than from anybody else—and they know it. But if they will be hounded for their bill they will never come near us. If we lose their good will too, they will make other enemies for us. I want them to hold their heads high when they come into my store, and to keep right on coming. That means, sometime, they will pay."

The result of this reasoning is that the druggist should transfer the account to losses, and tell his customer about it. He gives up the attempt to collect? Not at all. He continues selling this customer on credit? Not that either. Read letter #3 and see how it solves the whole problem and keeps the trade.

These suggestions for collecting accounts are humbly offered in the hope that they may be of help to you in what we believe is an unnecessary evil—retail charge accounts. It is gratifying to learn that during the past few years a great may of our stockholders have discontinued extending credit to their customers and adopted a strictly cash policy because they had sustained heavy losses on charge accounts, and further because the burden of carrying such accounts—which in some instances represented several thousand dollars—was more than they could stand if they were to remain in business. More retailers every year wake up to the folly of giving credit and determine to do business for CASH.

The chief objection to the adoption by everybody of the CASH system is the idea that "IT CAN'T BE DONE," but this is simply a mental attitude. The fact that it is the correct way and that IT IS BEING DONE successfully by a continually increasing majority of those dealing with the consumer, leads the retailer who has the courage of his convictions directly to the determination to SELL FOR CASH.

MILLIONS OF DOLLARS would be released for other and better uses if salaried men and others would arrange to have cash in hand to meet current expenses. If every farmer at the end of his crop year would lay aside the money to pay as he goes rather than get the credit at the store the difficulty could be solved. It simply means the exercise of foresight. That will solve the problem.

First Request

Dear Mr. _____

A considerable part of the amount on the enclosed statement is past due. Evidently you overlooked this last month.

I surely appreciate your trade and am always anxious to please you, not only by giving you the best possible service my store can offer, but also by extending credit to you whenever that makes buying more convenient for you. My prices, however, are all figured on a cash basis, so I must see that my book accounts never represent a large percentage of my investment in this business.

May I not expect to receive your check shortly?

Very truly yours,
[Account manager]

Second Request

Dear Mr. _____

On [date] I advised you of the amount which my books showed you to be owing at that time and I tried to impress upon you how necessary it was for me to have prompt settlements of all charge accounts.

I feel certain that you had intended to care for this matter promptly, but probably other things came up which caused you to overlook it, and now that you have this reminder before you, you will gladly see to it that this account is paid.

I shall plan on receiving your remittance within a day or two.

Yours very truly,

[Account manager]

Notice of Transfer to Doubtful Accounts

Dear Mr. _____

We are disappointed. We expected that you would find it possible to make payment to us on that old account before this time, and we are sorry indeed that our fine record of collections must be spoiled by charging this to "Losses on Accounts." Fortunately they have been very small so far, and we suppose there must have been some sad reason for your failure to pay up.

We have today closed your account by transferring it to our list of "Doubtful Accounts." This does not mean that we have given up hopes of collecting it. It simply means that we did not want it to appear "open" in our charge accounts hereafter.

We want you and your family to visit our store very often to see all the fine new things and the constantly increasing advantages which we are always offering. In these visits you will never be bothered with this unpaid account. That is for our office people to attend to, and as your account is now "closed" they will not send you any more "dunning letters" until your financial condition has improved.

It is our sincere wish that better times may come for you in the future, and we know that you will then be glad to remember and pay this old debt. It is always particularly pleasant when we receive payments on doubtful accounts that have been charged to "Losses." We feel sure that you will cause us this pleasure some time, hence, we will not worry about your account hereafter, but will try to serve you so well that we will always deserve and receive all, or a good share, of your trade in our lines.

Yours truly,

[Account manager]

Other letters, such as one numbered 329 (date undocumented), from H. L. Simpson, Sales Manager, told of new money-saving opportunities:

It's a Freight Prepaid offer on all your purchases of Family Remedies (Trailers), Puretest and Pharmaceuticals for January only. So we may start all together and early in 1923 to make the Year our BIGGEST OWN GOODS YEAR, your Company is making you an offer extraordinary that will demand the attention and receive the action of those who really want to make more net profits.

In another letter, dated May 1921, Simpson exhorted Rexallites to take stock of their sales. Who could resist his logic?

Dear Rexallite:

JUST WHAT ARE YOU GOING TO DO ABOUT IT?

If the enclosed card shows your purchases for the first three months of this year exceed those for the same period last year, are you going to keep that progressive step all to yourself, or are you going to let your sales people share in this knowledge of your further advancement in sound business policies?

If your sales people are not interested in the sale of your own controlled merchandise there can be but two reasons; either you haven't done your part to teach them why you want merchandise featured and sold that is manufactured by your Company in which you have money invested whose products stand for the HIGHEST IN QUALITY, the sale being confined exclusively in your town to your store, or when they have this knowledge which they are entitled to (and the sales people in the better Rexall stores possess these facts and more) and then do not respond, the wheels of elimination should start to grind, for no one can afford to carry dead-wood in his sales organization.

Should the card show your purchases are less, are you going to console yourself with the excuse that business is a little off? *Man, in Heaven's name,* if your business is off, doesn't that very condition demand a greater sale of Own Goods? Extra time and effort put forth right here means increased profits now and in the future.

Talk it over with your sales force. They will appreciate your suggestions. If you need merchandise to back up any sales campaign you may formulate, an order on the enclosed order blank will be greatly appreciated and demand our immediate attention.

After some fraudulent aspirin tablets, made by another firm, were discovered on the market, Rexallites were provided with six samples of ad copy to take advantage of the situation. Here is one:

THE ASPIRIN SITUATION

Don't Be Deceived by Aspirin advertisements being run by those who seek to discredit all Aspirin Tablets except those made by them.

The Facts Are that we regularly handle large quantities of Aspirin U. D. Co. Tablets that we know are Pure and Genuine. They are rigidly tested by first-class chemists and are put out by a firm of the very highest standing, the United Drug Company of Boston. We, as Rexall Druggists, are their exclusive agents in Tampa.

The Aspirin patent expired in 1917 and anyone can now make Aspirin and sell it under that name.

Aspirin U. D. Co. Tablets are put up in packages of 12's; 24's; 100's. The price is moderate, for there is no profiteering in the United Drug Co. Business methods.

TAYLOR DRUG COMPANY
TAMPA, FLORIDA

Surely it is now clear that Rexall was in every way—merchandising, promotion, debt collection—offering aid to their Rexall retailers. The phrase "Doing well by doing good" comes to mind, but that is not nearly the totality of Rexall efforts to encourage their customers to use approaches that worked.

CONVENTIONS AND TRAINING COURSES

For many of the early years, Rexall was small enough (although growth was phenomenal) to hold annual conventions for Rexallites. These conventions, at least in the early days, allowed a great deal of personal (family) interaction between corporate executives and Rexallites. They tended to be a combination of "good time is had by all" commercials for Rexall and educational programs on merchandising. (There were, of course, no sessions on pharmacology, chemistry, etc., but that is not why the Rexallites attended.)

The conventions were a tremendous success. They often had a carnival atmosphere, as reported in an earlier chapter, and Rexall covered all the bases. One big event early on was the "Peace Jubilee," the fifteenth annual convention. United arranged for a special train, "De-Luxe," from Chicago to Boston in August 1919. A private train (see Chapter 7) was arranged "exclusively for Rexallites" and provided

a large club car, where you may retire and enjoy that El Solara Cigar, and possibly—well, we don't like to say too much—but maybe? [Not politically correct today, but let's continue.] This we will have, with plenty of room for all, and in addition—"FOR MEN ONLY"—a very mysterious Pullman which you will be invited to visit, at least once, while en route.

Given the persuasiveness of this communication (reproduced only in part), it is not surprising that Rexall also had also to provide "Rules Governing Attendance" at the 1919 Peace Jubilee. The rules had nothing to do with behavior but, rather, were designed to limit attendance by "outsiders." So popular had the conventions become that, apparently, some Rexallites wished to involve (many) others in the fun. Ever mindful of the sensitivity of their Rexall family members, the company imposed the rules, but with a gentleness:

> During the last national Rexall meeting held in Boston (in 1916), the officers and department managers of the Company were greatly handicapped in their efforts to get acquainted with our stockholders, especially those from a distance and who were visiting the plant for the first time, by the presence of so large a number of *outsiders*. Without some restrictions we would doubtless have even more difficulty this year in confining the convention to the Rexall Family.

> The Committee is certain that no loyal Rexallite ever willfully disregarded the rights of his fellow stockholders by inviting outsiders to take part in entertainment which the Company provided for Rexallites only; but some have allowed themselves, in the past, to be imposed upon by their inconsiderate friends, and the United Drug Company and its legitimate guests have been the sufferers.

> This unpleasant subject is being frankly discussed because the Committee does not want any Rexallite to think that those whom *he* would like to bring are not welcome. The fact is, the Rexall Family is now so large that we are not able to provide for outsiders as we have in the past. It is not a question of *willingness* to entertain the friends of our stockholders; we simply cannot accomplish the impossible, and we are sure no reasonable Rexallite would ask us to attempt it.

> Regardless, therefore, of the Company's well-known hospitality, the following rules have been adopted, and *they must and will be rigidly enforced:*

> Each Rexall Store will be entitled to representation by one, two, or not more than three of the following persons: (a) the proprietor; or (b) one or more of the store owners; or (c) the manager; or (d) one or more of the store's salespeople.

These rules in no way dampened the enthusiasm for conventions, which continued as a major event for many years. Indeed, they became so successful, and Rexall grew so large, that national conventions gave way to regional and even state conventions.

The company prepared "Rexall-logues"—talks illustrated by motion pictures, one for each department in the store, at a cost of $100,000 each. These were made especially for conventions, even at the state level. At the 1921 Wisconsin Rexall Convention the subject was "Merchandising in the Rexall Store." The program, reprinted here, provides an example of how Rexall strove to help the Rexallites:

Tuesday Morning

8:00   Registration. Shaking hands with old and new friends.

9:00   Meeting of the General Convention Committee in Convention Hall.

10:00   Convention called to order by the President of the Wisconsin Rexall Club, R. L. Milbauer, Clintonville.

10:05   A Word of Welcome by Mr. H. C. Heffern, Manager Owl Drug Store, Milwaukee.

10:15   Greetings from the Home Office by H. L. Simpson, General Sales Manager, United Drug Company.

10:25   From this point on, the meeting, except four periods, will be devoted to the important subject of MERCHANDISING IN THE REXALL STORE IN YOUR TOWN, beginning with METHODS OF INCREASING VOLUME

1. Through Advertising.
   a. What percent of your volume should be spent on advertising? How should it be spent to produce results?
   b. The value of the various forms of Advertising, such as Rexall Magazine, Calendar, Almanac, Motion Picture Slides, Enclosure Strips, Novelties, Outdoor Advertising, etc. Where should each variety be used?
   c. Methods of distribution.
   d. Methods of backing up national advertising which will bring more volume to the store?
2. Through Service.
   a. What constitutes good service?
   b. Is good service a vital thing in a small town?

     c. Will good service contribute to building up and holding a business?

     d. How can employees be interested in giving good service?

  3. Through Displays.

     a. How should they be made?

     b. How to build floor displays that will sell?

     c. Use of bins, trays, etc., for displaying small items on counters?

     d. Use of price tickets and show cards?

     e. Value of your windows?

     f. Methods of store arrangement?

  4. Through Special Sales—Weekly, Monthly or Seasonable?
Candy
Hospital and Rubber
Toilet Goods
Puretest
Rexall and Riker Remedies
Sundries
Food Products
Stationery
One-Cent Sales
Week End Sales

  5. Through Getting the Doctor's Business at a Profit, Also
Hospitals
Institutions
Schools
Manufacturing Plants
Offices, etc.

12:25   Announcements

12:30   Adjournment for luncheon as guests of the Rexall Clubs

Tuesday Afternoon

2:00   Rexall-logue on Candy. This will be a talk on the production of Candy illustrated by motion pictures, beginning with the cocoa plantations of Trinidad and carrying the audience in a brief way through the gathering and preparing of cocoa beans. It will cover in detail all phases of the manufacturing of chocolate products and candy as conducted at your own plants, the Chocolate Refiners Company of Mansfield, Mass., and the United Candy Company, Boston, Mass.

3:25   Candy. Short talk by H. W. Taylor, Manager of the Department, followed by a general discussion.

4:25   Appointment of Nominating Committee.

4:30   Announcements.

4:35   Adjourn.

Tuesday Evening

8:00   Theatre Party tendered by the United Drug Company.

Wednesday Morning

9:30   Rexall-logue on Rubber and Hospital. An illustrated talk covering the production of all rubber goods, from the gathering of crude rubber in Brazil and India, through the manufacturing processes as conducted at your own Seamless Rubber Company, New Haven, and the proper methods of displaying and selling in Rexall Stores.

10:55   Toilet Goods Department. Short talk by Miss Mae I. Nellgan, Perfume Department, Boston, followed by a general discussion.

11:50   What shall be done with the State Bonus Fund?

12:00   METHODS OF INCREASING GROSS PROFIT

1. Through Pushing the Long Profit Line.
    a. How it can be done without offending the customer
    b. Taking advantage of the universal guarantee
    c. Proper methods of displaying and advertising the line
    d. Commission plans that work and do not require extra detail

12:25   Announcements.

12:30   Adjournment for luncheon as guests of the Rexall Clubs.

Wednesday Afternoon

2:00   METHODS OF INCREASING GROSS PROFIT—*Continued.*

2. Through Use of the Bulletin Board.
    a. How to stimulate concentration on any item or list of items
    b. How to double net profits through use of the bulletin board
    c. Stimulating sales by setting a quota

3. Through Stock Standardization.
   a. Easy methods of taking inventory
   b. Keeping stock up and investment down
   c. Increasing turnover
4. Through Methods of Handling Accounts.
   a. Collections
   b. Taking discounts
   c. Making use of local bank

4:30   Election and Installation of Officers.

4:45   A Parting Message from Mr. Simpson.

5:00   Final Adjournment.

Wednesday Evening

7:00   Banquet tendered by United Drug Company. Music, songs and entertainment. A good time for everybody.

Ultimately, the number of Rexallites became too large for conventions, so other means of communication became necessary. The "Rexall Train," described in Chapter 7, was one incredible example. Another was the Rexall course in business training. Here is an edited version of how it was described to potential enrollees.

SCOPE OF THE COURSE

The Rexall Course consists of eighteen lessons, each printed in good clear type in handy pocket size. The subjects covered by the course are:

Book 1. Business and Salesmanship Fundamentals.
Books 2 and 3. How to develop Personal Efficiency.
Book 4. Sizing Up the Customer.
Book 5. Drug Store Service.
Book 6. Business Efficiency in the Drug Store.
Book 7. Advertising, Letter Writing and the Telephone.
Book 8. Store Management and Sales Methods.
Book 9. How to Study Goods.
Book 10. How to Sell Rexall Remedies.
Book 11. How to Sell Perfumery and Toilet Preparations.
Book 12. How to Sell Stationery and School Supplies.
Book 13. How to Sell Candy.
Book 14. The Soda Fountain.
Book 15. How to Sell Rubber Goods and Hospital Supplies.

Book 16. How to Sell Cigars and Tobacco.
Book 17. The Prescription and Bulk Drug Department.
Book 18. Publicity.

THE CERTIFICATE OF MERIT

These titles merely suggest the range of vital subjects covered. Questions testing the student's understanding are in each book and their answers are graded and commented upon. Students attaining satisfactory grades secure a special diploma. This diploma is issued by the College of Business Administration of Boston University and bears the signature of President Louis K. Liggett as well as those of Secretary Thos. V. Wooten of the International Association of Rexall Clubs, Prof. Whitehead and Dean Lord of the College of Business Administration.

HOW THE WORK IS CONDUCTED

Prof. Harold Whitehead, head of the Department of Sales Relations of Boston University, wrote the course and personally conducts it. Mr. Wooten collaborated with Professor Whitehead thus insuring a course admirably adapted to the day-in and day-out requirements of the Rexall Store. . . .

COST OF THE COURSE

The Rexall Course is sold below cost to Rexallites and their clerks. No on else can buy it at any price.

The price is only $15.00 and will be charged to the Rexallite's account in the usual way. This price is subject to change without notice. A new printing will soon be necessary when the price *must* be advanced.

Enroll today. A lesson will be mailed to you every two weeks.

The course is sold to you on the Rexall Guarantee—money back if you are not satisfied with the benefits which it brings to you and the store in which you work.

Clerk Training

Speaking of education, a true piece of genius was Rexall's emphasis on and assistance in clerk training. Training conventions were held at no cost to the Rexallite except the cost of travel. Here is how the concept was introduced in 1920.

Clerks

Dear Rexallite:

If your drug store is like the average, your clerks ring the cash register oftener than you do. Each ringing by them ought to bring you the feeling: "Another satisfied customer has contributed his daily quota to the store's success." Does it produce that feeling? Are you confident the customer is satisfied? Will he surely come back? Did he make as many purchases as he might and buy the goods best suited to him and most profitable to the store?

At your Club's last meeting the quest of clerks' meetings was discussed at length and the officers were instructed to do whatever they thought best. After carefully studying the subject from every viewpoint, especially the experiences of other progressive Rexall clubs, these officers decided that in no other way could the Club's Bonus Fund be spent to such good advantage.

The enclosed program of the convention to be held Tuesday and Wednesday, March 16-17, in Chicago, will show you that for two days the young men and women in attendance will devote their entire time to discussing, under the direction of the United Drug Company's Officers and Department Managers, the problems hourly presenting themselves in every Rexall store. Let us consider a few of the benefits, which these officers believe this meeting will bring to your clerks:

How to make the windows pull people into the store; how to arrange inside-the-store displays which will sell goods; how to be real salesmen instead of waiters; how to make companion sales; how to keep customers from trading at competitors' stores. Among other things it will give him or her: A better knowledge of the United Drug Company; first-hand information as to how our own controlled products are manufactured; a good understanding of what the International Rexall Movement means; praiseworthy ambition to be real drug merchants instead of mere "drug clerks."

To reap the benefits of this meeting all you have to do is to buy your clerk a round-trip ticket, give him or her money for one or two breakfasts, also for supper the last evening. The other expenses, including room at the hotel for one night, will be paid by the several Rexall Clubs which are participating and the United Drug Company. If you want to send more than one responsible clerk, we'll be glad to have both or even three. Don't fail to have it plainly understood, though, that this is not an outing but a business investment from which you expect good returns.

If the young man (or woman) you send is really interested in his work, we feel sure the increased knowledge and the new enthusiasm he brings home with him will cause him to ring the cash register oftener, and when he does you will have confidence that no opportunities on your behalf have been neglected. These clerks' meetings have had just that effect wherever they've been tried. That we may make badges and know how many to secure rooms for, be sure to sign and return the enclosed card at once.

Example of Work of "Clubs"

One of the officers of the Wisconsin Upper Michigan Rexall Club urged his fellow Rexallites to see the value of such programs:

Dear Rexallite:

Secretary Wooten's recent letter brought out forcibly what I had thought of before—the absurdity of employing clerks instead of salespeople when clerks, because they fail to use the opportunities they are provided with, cost *a great deal more,* in spite of the fact that their salaries may be less.

Said I to myself: "What's the use of advertising to bring people INTO the store if use is not made of the buying attitude of these customers when they get there?" And then I got to wondering whether it's my own fault if my employees fail to measure up in the matter of salesmanship ability. Have I helped them as I ought? Whatever the answer, the resolution I formed was this: "I am going to send to the convention in Madison, Thursday, Oct. 9th, also in Green Bay, Monday, Oct. 13th, just as many of my own boys and girls as I can possibly spare and I am going to urge my fellow Rexallites to do likewise."

A hard-headed businessman who understands human nature and knows what we druggists are up against said to me not long ago: "Druggists could have better help in their stores if they were not so short-sighted. They employ a new clerk, tell him a few things about their business (but almost nothing), then they watch to see whether he gets the results they want. If he doesn't produce, they fire him on the first or second payday and hire another. They treat him the same way with the same outcome. Then they growl about what they call 'hard luck' but what looks to me a good deal like lack of common sense. As far as my observation goes, they all act the same way. How on earth is a clerk to learn to be a salesman if somebody along the line doesn't take the time and trouble to teach him?"

Of course, I didn't tell that fellow how near he came to guessing the truth; but can we deny that in the case of a great many druggists he hit the nail squarely on the head? Now, then, when the United Drug Company goes to the expense of arranging for these salespeople's conventions, sending some of their best men to attend them, how foolish it would be for us not to use this opportunity of having SOME of this work of training taken off our hands by those who know so well how to do it?

Let's all go in and help to make this meeting a big success. It will not cost any of us very much (just the railroad fare of our people) and we will all regard the outlay a mere pittance in comparison with the big results of having new life and a better spirit put into those who contribute so largely to our business success. That we may know how many to get ready for, please sign and return the enclosed card, and *do it now*. Thank you.

Clerks were not just exposed to sales training; their opinions were sought. In one mailing, they were offered the opportunity to submit "Questions I'd Like to Have Answered at the Coming Rexall Clerks' Convention." They were challenged to put their advancing skills to work at the convention. Here is the contest offered to "Junior Rexallites":

Dear Junior Rexallite:

If a customer asked you for Zinc Ointment, you would probably sell him several other articles besides. What would these articles be, supposing you had no other "lead"? You have *your* ideas of what ought to be offered him; your fellow clerks have *theirs*. The same is true of other often-called-for articles. Whoever submits the best list of companion items, as indicated herein, will pocket the First Prize—$15.00; the second best list will pull down the Second Prize—$10.00; the third best list will draw the Third Prize—$5.00.

The "best" list will be adjudged to be such for the following reasons: First, because of the Suitableness of the additional items. (Are the items such as can be used to advantage in conjunction with the article called for and has the customer been benefitted by your selling them to him?) Secondly, because of the benefits the store will get from the standpoint of Profit and

Repeat Business. (Do the items give the store ample profit and, if they are satisfactory to the customer, will he return to *your* store—the Rexall Store—for more instead of going to some other drug store?)

In order to compete, all you have to do is to fill out the blank below and bring it to the Convention. The lists will be collected the first day and the prizes awarded at the Banquet that night.

* * *

Dear Mr. Secretary: If a customer asked me for one of the items on the top line, below, I would endeavor to sell him the other items which I have placed in the column below it.

My name is _____

Of the Rexall Store of _____

Date: _____, 1921

Located at _____

Zinc Ointment	Sugar of Milk	Shaving Lotion	A Hair Brush	Hot Water Bottle	Bella-donna Plaster	Tooth Paste	Razor Strop	Cold Tablets

REXALL AD-VANTAGES

Almost from the beginning, United Drug began publishing *Rexall Ad-Vantages*. It was described on the masthead as "A Magazine of Get Together" and published by the Advertising Department.

Rexall Ad-Vantages often ran to fifty or more pages in a large 9½" × 13½" magazine format. It was a combination of several elements, but the primary mission was to provide Rexallites with scores of merchandising ideas in every issue. One reason for its success, and part of its genius, was that many of the ideas came from Rexallites themselves. Thus, the magazine featured individual involvement from druggists who got the chance to see their names in print. *Always* a good idea.

The magazine included news and detailed reports from every convention, as well as success stories, cartoons, some occasional philosophy, and announcements of new products. Readers were provided with sample newspaper ads, window displays, and hypothetical problems that were followed the next month by suggested solutions. An example of the kind of pithy advice given by Rexallites to their fellow druggists was this from an Indiana pharmacist in 1912:

> Most large drug stores employ young lady clerks at the Toilet Goods Counter. But though we believe that this is done by very few stores in towns of five thousand population or less, our experience proves that *every* Rexall Store, whether large or small, should employ a young lady clerk.
>
> This young lady should be popular, neat in her dress, and an intelligent talker. We selected a girl who had studied a year in college, who was a fraternity member and very popular, and who, having always lived in Franklin, was well acquainted with the people. She had two years' mercantile experience in a high-class gift store, and was very anxious to join our sales force.
>
> After she had been in the store two weeks, had learned about toilet goods, stationery and cigar stocks, and had caught the Rexall enthusiasm, we mailed, by first-class postage, three hundred correspondence cards to a carefully selected list of women. The cards were signed by the girl and the envelopes were addressed by her, and we daily note gratifying results from this distribution.
>
> We believe that during the holidays this girl will prove to be a wonder at "suggestive salesmanship." Women like to buy their toilet and stationery articles from a girl whom they like, who knows her business and who can suggest the newest and best things. Men, too, like to buy their cigars from a fresh, bright-faced young girl. We are absolutely sure that it pays to employ women in the drug store.

What a revolutionary idea!

United also found a way to make money through *Ad-Vantages,* by accepting advertising from other firms (e.g., for typewriters, as noted in Chapter 5). They were careful to point out, however, the policy behind the inclusion of ads.

> The columns of *Ad-Vantages* are open to a very carefully selected list of outside advertisers.
>
> To the stockholders of the United Drug Company we wish to announce that while we do not stand as sponsor for any of these firms, nor wish to be held responsible in any misunderstandings or disputes which could by chance arise between any of them and any of our stockholders, yet we have not and will not, in a single instance, accept any advertisement until we have proved that the firm behind it is entirely responsible and reputable and their goods dependable. In this direction we desire to afford our stockholders all the protection possible, and at the same time we hope they will, whenever quality and price is at least equal, show their appreciation of the patronage that advertisers in *Ad-Vantages* are giving them by extending their patronage to them, whenever convenient.
>
> We assure you these advertisers would not be represented in the advertising pages of *Ad-Vantages* if there was any doubt in our minds about their dependability.

Rexall also began publishing, in 1912, *The Rexall News,* later changed to *The Rexall Magazine*. It was aimed at the female consumer, and while it contained plenty of ads for Rexall products, these were interspersed with puzzles, recipes, jokes, and stories. In 1913 Rexallites could purchase as few as five hundred copies for $4.50. They were allowed their own imprint on the front and back and a choice of six ads for the back cover each month.

In 1956 *The Rexall Reporter* was launched. This was more a news magazine for Rexallites, designed to keep them informed of Rexall promotional activities and also, as before, to highlight successes of franchisees. It was light on advice for success.

THE SALES FORCE

Rexall was, of course, represented by a nationwide team of salespeople whose job was to call on Rexall druggists, generate orders,

and provide merchandising assistance. Two years of some kind of retail experience were required before you could get a job in Rexall
sales (PC 73). Once hired, the recruit received a full year of formal
training, along with a book of instructions on which he was tested.
(This particular respondent [PC 73] was assigned the responsibility
of the Christmas trunk show for his area. This involved hauling forty-
eight steamer trunks of merchandise, by train, to set up a trade show
for Rexall druggists.)

THE FRANCHISES

By the 1950s Rexall had nine distribution centers in the United
States and three in Canada. The exact number of franchisees varied,
but in 1954 Rexall reported just over 10,000 in the United States and
another 1,400 in Canada. The franchise arrangement, still the heart
and soul of Rexall, was originally of three kinds, with a fourth added
later:

> *White:* Issued to the original stockholders and some early cus-
> tomers. Signed by Liggett himself.
> *Blue:* Covered a whole (small) town
> *Pink:* Necessary for large cities and included street boundaries,
> such as south of High Street between Fifteenth and Thirty-
> Fourth Streets (Of course, preventing "seepage" was diffi-
> cult.)
> *Orange:* The last issued

A sample franchise agreement is reproduced in the photograph
section of this book, but easy-to-understand reasons for becoming a
franchisee are provided in two Rexall brochures. The first is *18 Most-
Asked Questions About Rexall:*

1. **Why should I sign a Rexall Franchise now?**
   The sooner you become a Rexall Druggist, the sooner you increase your volume and profit. The Rexall Franchise is the
   quickest way to relieve your business headaches. The cost of
   doing business has skyrocketed. Rents and wages are up, yet
   prices on drug store merchandise are down because of intensive competition between brands, supermarkets and other
   local retailers. Only Rexall can relieve your business head-

aches for you. Rexall provides you Quality drug products with a higher gross profit—products which are exclusively yours—Preplanned Promotions, National Advertising, Store Identification, Point-of-Sale Kits and Local Advertising Aids.

2. What Profits will I make on Rexall products?
The gross profit on Rexall products averages approximately 50 percent throughout the line. As you know, this is much higher than the gross profit you are now making on your merchandise.

3. What proof is there that Rexall's margins are better than competition's?
Rexall eliminates the middleman. As a result, you are buying direct from our laboratories. This, plus the mass buying power of 10,000 Rexall druggists, makes Rexall gross profits higher. Surveys by a nationally known research company show, for example, that on your sales of alkalizers—all brands—you average 17.1 percent gross profit, while Rexall's Bisma Rex provides you 53 percent. On aspirin—all brands—you average 26.9 percent gross profit, while Rexall Aspirin would provide you 59.2 percent. And so it goes with all Rexall products.

4. Are Rexall products asked for by brand name like other nationally advertised merchandise?
Yes. Through many years of national advertising, the public has been educated that Rexall products can be purchased only at a Rexall Drug Store. As a result, the public specifically asks for Rexall products at Rexall Drug Stores.

5. What is the best-known name in drugs?
Rexall. A recent survey shows that five times as many people named Rexall over other drug products when asked, "Who do you think of *first* in drugs?" The same survey also shows that five times as many people mentioned Rexall as the first name that comes to mind when thinking of drug stores.

6. Is Rexall a developer of new products?
Yes. At Rexall Research Laboratories in Los Angeles, hundreds of specialists are continually developing new products, as well as improving existing products. Rexall research keeps in touch with all parts of the world for new developments. Since Rexall products are manufactured in Rexall laboratories, superior quality control can be enforced.

7. Is Rexall a "House" line of merchandise?

Yes, in a sense, and this is good. Rexall offers a complete line of high gross drug products that are sold exclusively at Rexall Drug Stores. Customers must return to your Rexall store to get this popular merchandise. Rexall gives you one brand throughout your store to recommend to your customers. And, as you know, every Rexall product contains a complete "Money-Back Guarantee."

8. What promotional assistance does Rexall offer?

Rexall offers a complete year-around promotional program. It is based on five major sale events, including two One-Cent Sales, and is supported by many in-store departmental drives throughout the year. The Rexall druggist has the most complete promotional activity in the drug retailing business. His promotional effort is backed by national advertising, local advertising aids, and point-of-sale material that give the maximum effect, with a minimum amount of effort on his part.

9. How much profit do I make on Rexall One-Cent Sale merchandise?

You make 60 percent gross profit on all One-Cent Sale merchandise, except during the twelve-day period of the two One-Cent Sales. On these days, you make 20 percent. You can sell Rexall One-Cent Sale merchandise all year around.

10. When do I have the opportunity to buy One-Cent Sale merchandise ?

You can buy One-Cent Sale merchandise nine months out of the year.

11. How does Rexall advertising make me a national advertiser?

Rexall's national advertising is "retail" advertising for your Rexall store. Its advertising is much the same as you would do yourself. It appears in your local Sunday newspaper and on your local television station, yet has the advantage of the prestige and consumer acceptance of national advertising. Rexall advertising also appears in many national magazines.

12. Is it true that I only have to pay 2½ percent of my Rexall purchases for Rexall national advertising?

Yes. Your share of Rexall national advertising cannot exceed 2½ percent of your purchases from Rexall. Rexall more than matches your 2½ percent for your national advertising program, to more than double the amount of advertising. Your cost would average approximately ¼ of 1 percent of your total volume.

13. How much will it cost me to add Rexall identification?

Identification costs vary according to the physical construction of your building. You have already seen, or will shortly see, a selection of proposals for the identification of your store. Any one of these proposals is what we recommend to enable you to cash in on Rexall's name. This cost will be financed for you at no charge over a convenient period of time.

14. How large an initial order of Rexall merchandise must I buy?

There is no set amount. Rexall only requires a representative stock of Rexall merchandise, so that you can back up Rexall's nationally advertised promotions and take care of the demands created by this advertising.

15. Do I have to buy merchandise I don't think will sell?

No, you are a better judge of what you can sell in your store than Rexall. But experience has shown us that all nationally advertised Rexall merchandise does move, and it would be unwise not to take advantage of this powerful selling aid.

16. Do I have to take on a large duplicate inventory when I take on Rexall?

No, Rexall does not want you to create excessive inventories on any product. You should buy only enough to back up the national advertising. Then when your existing stock depletes, you will want to replace with Rexall merchandise because of Rexall's higher gross profit.

17. What is the public opinion of a store that switches to Rexall?

Surveys show that, in the minds of your customers, the moment your store becomes a Rexall store, your service increases 25 percent, your quality increases 37 percent and your prices are 44 percent lower.

18. Will I lose my identity when I switch to Rexall?

No, the marriage of Rexall to your local respected name will bring you increased volume and profits. It will join the two most important names in the drug business—your own locally respected name and Rexall's nationally respected name—giving you a combination that can't be beat.

The second pamphlet, issued in 1960, was titled *What Rexall Can Do for You:*

The Cost of Doing Business Is Up— More Intensive Competition

Rent, wages and fixed costs are up. Plus more and more outlets are selling your drug store products, especially supermarkets, national firms and other local retailers. You have confusion and competition among suppliers who see you as but a small part of their picture.

There Is a Prescription to Relieve These Problems

This prescription requires three rare ingredients:

1. Higher gross profit on each unit of sale.
2. Exclusive merchandise that will bring you repeat business.
3. A planned promotional program to increase your volume.

Rexall Fills 10,000 of These Prescriptions Every Day

Rexall fills these prescriptions with:

High Quality Drug Products with a higher gross profit that are exclusive at Rexall Drug Stores
Preplanned storewide and departmental Promotions
National Advertising
Store Identification
Point-of-Sale Kits
Local Advertising Aids

Rexall Means High Quality Drug Products with a Higher Gross Profit

Rexall has a team of research scientists and new products experts developing the newest and best in drug store products. These products are manufactured in Rexall's modern mass production laboratories which maintain the high standards of production and quality control. And in addition, Rexall gives you superior packaging which is the best in design and salability. A few examples of Rexall's quality drug products are Bisma-Rex, Super Anapac, Thru and Super Plenamins, which is America's largest selling vitamin-mineral product.

Rexall products are sold to franchised retailers only, at prices which provide you with a higher gross profit. The price to retailers is the same in every state. Rexall customers know they can find Rexall's exclusive products at a fair price at Rexall stores everywhere.

Rexall Means Preplanned Promotions

All through the year Rexall boosts your sales with preplanned promotions, both storewide and departmental, to move not only Rexall products, but all merchandise in your store. They include the famous One-Cent Sale, which is the most effective promotion in drug retailing history.

Rexall Means National Advertising

Network Television, National Magazine, and Newspaper advertising give Rexall Drug Stores a national reputation that when combined with your local reputation makes an unbeatable combination. Presently Rexall national advertising uses network television and newspaper ads in your local Sunday newspaper to give tremendous impact to Rexall's nationwide promotions. Other ads in national magazines back individual promotions behind new and exclusive Rexall products.

Rexall Means Store Identification

In order to let people know that you have the products that are nationally advertised, it is important that your store is identified with the Rexall Orange and Blue. No matter where people are from, the Rexall sign is a familiar one, standing for quality, reliability, clean, well-lighted stores and friendly service.

Rexall Means Point-of-Sale Material

Once inside your drug store, Rexall point-of-sale material lets your customers know that you have the merchandise they have seen advertised. Once a month you receive beautifully lithographed counter cards, window cards, price tickets, and reprints, banners, etc., for

Rexall promotions and other special occasions like Valentine's Day, Easter, and Back-to-School.

Rexall Means Local Advertising Aids

Your name will be imprinted on major promotion circulars. Newspaper mats, TV and radio commercials, filmed and live scripts, calendars and almanacs are some of the local advertising material available. These aids bring the national advertising down to your local level. They let your customers know where to buy locally what they have seen advertised nationally.

The Rexall Plan Means $ucce$$

The Rexall Plan as outlined on the preceding pages has been developed and refined over the last fifty-seven years. As a result, the 10,000 Rexall Drug Stores that are following this plan are making more money.

These stores are doing 30 percent of the retail drug business though they number only 17 percent of all the drug stores in the United States.

And they average 30 percent more volume than non-Rexall drug stores because they follow the Rexall Plan.

Rexall Means Progress

Because Rexall means progress, the moment you become a Rexall store, in the minds of your customers, your quality increases 37 percent, your service increases 25 percent, and your prices are 44 percent lower. At least that's what customers told us in a recent impartial survey.

In a national consumer survey, when asked, "Who do you think of first in drugs?"—five times as many people named Rexall over other drug products.

And five times as many people, when thinking of drug stores, thought of Rexall first.

WHY DON'T YOU?

WHOLESALING

Although Rexall bypassed the wholesaler with its own Rexall products, thus providing larger profit margins for its franchisees, there were plenty of non-Rexall products sold in these drugstores. To help them in acquiring these products, the United Wholesale Druggists was formed as a subsidiary. This was a co-op of retailers headquartered in Boston, but with distribution centers geographically dispersed. The co-op was discontinued in 1956 (PC 73).

CONCLUSION

It worked! The partnership worked—because of the genius infused into it by Liggett and his team.

Chapter 7

The Genius of Rexall Promotion

Although much can be said about Rexall promotion, let's start with the story of one of the most outrageous, extraordinary, attention-getting promotional schemes of the twentieth century.

THE REXALL TRAIN

In 2000, the Terminal Railroad Association of St. Louis Historical and Technical Society published, under the able editorship of Larry Thomas, a forty-three-page monograph titled *The Rexall Story.*[1] The heart of it was the story of the Rexall Train, but much attention is given to Rexall itself. The author of the current book would be a fool not to rely heavily on this reference (although accounts of the train appear elsewhere) so here I acknowledge my debt to this publication.

Here are Larry Thomas's words describing the train's first stop, in St. Louis, destined to be the final resting place of Rexall (sort of):

> Lettering across the top of the tender reads New York Central, but the streamlined sheet metal on the locomotive attracts the most interest. No one has seen anything like it before. The locomotive [see the picture section] is entirely streamlined with the metal configured to project smooth flowing lines. The metal work driving wheels on both sides bear a sign that reads "The Rexall Train." (p. 18)

Louis Liggett, faced with the difficulty of getting all of his Rexall druggists to conventions, decided to bring Rexall to them. Before its adventure was over, the Rexall Train visited over 100 cities on a 29,000-mile journey. Where did Liggett get the idea? That's not clear, although Liggett had seen the streamliner Commodore Vanderbilt, which was "sleek and fast" and reportedly called the president of New York Central Railroad shortly thereafter. As Thomas puts it, "once an idea was planted into Mr. Liggett's mind that promoted Rexall there was no turning back" *(Rexall Story)*.

It was reported that United Drug paid a million dollars for the special twelve-car train put together by the Pullman Company to trail the phenomenal locomotive. The train was stocked with Rexall merchandise and staffed by both Rexall employees (two pharmacists, a nurse, two Rexall women to distribute samples) and Pullman employees (engineers, porters, waiters, and chefs).

The journey started, appropriately, at headquarters in Boston (see the map in the picture section). Thousands of people visited the train en route—15,000 in Cincinnati alone. In Moberly, Missouri, with a population of only 16,000, some 8,200 boarded the Rexall Train. All along the route, of course, Rexall druggists were alerted in advance so that they could build the event into their store promotions—"free tickets" being a key element.

Various cars in the train bore their own names. The first two cars focused on Rexall products. "Kantleak" was named after Rexall's Two-in-One Stopperless Hot Water Bottle. It followed directly behind the locomotive and was a service center for the train. Next came "First Aid," named for Rexall's line of bandages and such and served the crew and staff. The remaining cars were more interesting.

The third car in the train was called "Ad-Vantages" after the in-house publication. Ad-Vantages and the following three cars were open to the public. During each stop the public had an opportunity to view displays, and Rexall druggists to hear lectures on merchandising and forthcoming products. One evening was reserved for dining and dancing. Ad-Vantages used displays and mirrors to create the illusion of a fully stocked drugstore. It *did* include a completely stocked soda fountain—a big hit!

The next car, "Research," contained a half-inch scale model of United's Research Department in Boston. The public (and Rexallites) could get an idea of the laboratory and testing activities, and local Rexallites could cite the educational value for youngsters.

"Bisma-Rex" was the next public car and featured Rexall's superstar product. It was, of course, a stomach antacid and, similar to some of its competitors, found inspiration in the success of Bromo-Seltzer, a product that, it was finally pointed out, had dangerous side effects.

"Cara-Nome," Rexall's brand of cosmetics, was the name given to the next public car. Of course it was filled with stylish showcases displaying the Cara-Nome line as well as an on-duty lady's cosmetics consultant offering grooming tips and samples. Rather incongruous, but very popular, was a display of the seven steps in making chocolate. Women and children, especially, left laden with samples, flyers, brochures, and other keepsakes—and terrific goodwill toward Rexall.

"Klenzo," the next car, was for Rexall druggists only and named after Rexall's line of bathroom products, toothpaste, and the like. This car was used as a lecture hall, seating eighty-eight by day, but could be cleared for dancing in the evening to music by the Rexall Orchestra.

"Symphony" was the dining car for Rexallites. Lunch and dinner were served by train staff. According to Thomas (*Rexall Story,* p. 31), "Pheasant on toast, broiled lobster tail in butter sauce and baked Virginia glazed ham were served on a whim." Pretty heady stuff for a small-town druggist! If the way to a man's heart is through his stomach, one cannot help but believe that it's a good way, also, to get to his order books.

"Adrienne," another lecture car, was followed by "Mi31," named after a product that was at one time, according to Thomas, the most popular mouthwash in the country. This was a lounge car with a full bar and dance floor. The four cars just described could accommodate, train, and educate hundreds during a single visit.

"Joan Manning," named for a not-very-successful line of chocolates, was next, and bringing up the rear was "Puretest," named after a large line of vitamins and what druggists called "wets and drys" (Epsom salts, rubbing alcohol, etc.). This is where Liggett himself traveled. It was a true executive facility as befitted a man of vision and substance and allowed him to host small private dinners and meals, and perhaps sign up another franchisee or two.

There was talk of a repeat train trip in 1937, but for a variety of reasons that never happened. Nevertheless, for one incredible year, Liggett took his traveling convention/carnival to forty-seven of the (then) forty-eight states to resounding success.

What did happen in 1937 was an extraordinary coincidence that perhaps foreshadowed the future of Rexall. Walgreens, Rexall's major competitor, acquired a *plane,* a six-passenger Lockheed Skydart. It was used for two years in much the same way as the Rexall Train, stopping in towns with Walgreens stores, giving free rides to customers, and generally spreading goodwill. Who was one of the pilots of the Skydart? None other than Justin Dart, soon to be appointed general manager of Walgreens.

REXALL PROMOTION FROM THE BEGINNING

From the outset, Liggett and his staff not only used every trick in the promotional book but also wrote new chapters. The early days featured a man with forty "believers," maybe a single product, and a vision. Think of the challenges Liggett faced as he set out to establish a national company. Promotion was essential to selling, but the media were limited—window displays, letters, billboards, flyers, posters, and similar items. Radio was not an option, and certainly not television. Even Liggett probably would not have believed in that possibility.

Thus, it was absolutely essential that druggists at the local level conduct vigorous promotional programs. Getting that to happen was part of the Liggett genius of the early days. One could not sit by and hope that those druggists would come up, individually, with effective promotional activities. (Of course some did.) Liggett and his staff instead supplied Rexallites with a variety of tools to build a promotional edifice, to encourage participation, and to provide inspiration.

The genius of Rexall promotion consisted of at least three parts:

1. In the early years, especially, the company provided their Rexall druggists with an avalanche of materials suitable for local promotion.
2. When national campaigns became possible, the company provided Rexallites with opportunities to "tie in" local promotions with national promotional efforts.
3. Finally, and perhaps most important, Rexall found ways to include the druggists themselves in national promotions. They

weren't just selling products; they were selling the people who offered those products to the public. Surely, this must have engendered a sense of pride and "ownership" in those Rexall druggists who took their partnership role seriously.

Initially Rexall promotion was, of necessity, through local channels. Dear Pardner letters, letters from other Rexall staffers, and *Rexall Ad-Vantages* were the primary media of promotion. *Rexall Ad-Vantages* was discussed in the previous chapter but deserves additional attention here.

Rexall Ad-Vantages

Within months after the company was founded, United Drug began publishing *Rexall Ad-Vantages.* As noted before, the publication offered a deluge of promotional ideas. It should be borne in mind that these Rexall druggists had no formal training in merchandising, and they needed (and presumably valued) the help offered by Rexall.

Besides sample ads, examples of window displays, and proposed letters to customers, the magazine offered regular written lessons in more depth. Some examples from the early days include the following:

- What to Spend for Ads, and How to Make the Investment Pay (by United's ad manager)
- Making the Fountain Pay
- Both Sides of the Counter—A Selling Talk
- Perfumes: Their History and Merchandising Possibilities
- Swat the Fly: A Big Plan Whereby You Can Turn a Public Liability into a Private Asset (a fly swatter sales promotion)
- Reaching the Public (by the assistant advertising manager)

Ad-Vantages included "pep talks" as well. The one that follows, though very long, is too good not to share. It is an editorial by Walter Jones Wilson from the January 1913 issue. Sure, it probably wouldn't work today, but it helps to show how hard Rexall worked to build team spirit.

Editorial

The cover design of this month's AD-VANTAGES is clever. Yet a captious critic could have a bit of fun with it. The artist pictures the power of co-operation applied to business. To do that he takes liberties with the laws of physics, astronomy and geography. Co-operation is likened to the sun illumining the earth. But the sun is 93,000,000 miles away, and any Rexall Druggist knows that co-operation is closer than that. To show how the light of a new intelligence is diffused in both hemispheres, the artist boldly moves Europe a few thousand miles westward nearer the American continent. But, even so, the picture does not show the old world and the new *as close together as they actually are drawn by this new power in business.*

What appears to be a moth ball punched through a target is the planet Saturn. At first I could not imagine why it was lugged into the picture. Then I remembered that as an ancient god Saturn presided over the work of seed sowing. So Saturn is accounted for. Down at the right a meteor blazes through space. It is meant, perhaps, to suggest the way the United Drug Company's progress looks to the outsider.

We know that the growth of the Rexall Idea has been logical, effect following cause in unbroken sequence; but the great thought, thus calmly accepted, flashed upon the world's eye ten years ago, splitting the darkness of misunderstanding and intolerance with a great white light. To us the glow is steady, revealing the way to better things. In the mind of "the man in the street," though, that first comparison lingers.

The attitude of this same average citizen toward the tremendous enterprise of which you are a part, his instinctive tribute of respect, holds a lesson for us.

We think we know what the Rexall proposition means. We talk glibly about it. In unwise moments we even boast of it. But do we—do *you*—really know what membership in the United Drug Company offers in the way of opportunity, what it entails in obligations?

It is no idle boast that Rexall Druggists are picked men. To be a picked man means that in the opinion of your fellow-workers you are a progressive; you have the spirit of leadership. From the very moment when to you is granted the privilege of calling your place of business The Rexall Store, you have ceased to be what you were. You may have been the most successful merchant in your locality, yesterday, seizing every opportunity as it came, but today *you, yourself, are Opportunity.* You have the purse of Fortunatus, the armor of Achilles.

Best of all, you have the spiritual backing of 5,000 good citizens of the world. Do not smile at that. One need not be a frantic metaphysician to realize that thought is a force; that the kindly wish, the collective hope of a man's friends for his well-being is a positive power shaping his progress. That great force is back of you, 5,000-fold. Five thousand keen minds are thinking of your commercial problems, 5,000 hands reach out to you in fellowship, 10,000 eyes watch your every move, smiling when you do well, filled with regret when you fail. Man, do you realize how weighty is your lightest act? Do you know that once a member of a world-wide fraternal order, such as the United Drug Company, you can never again live for yourself alone; that you have become personally responsible for the success of every one of your co-workers?

By a simple pen stroke you have merged your destiny with that of kindred spirits in far countries.

You have endorsed the note of progress.

In accepting the responsibility of a Rexall Druggist you have said to the world, "I will live true to the vow of service. As you find my brothers worthy of trust, so shall you find me." Alone, the task, though voluntarily assumed, would be arduous. But how glorious is the thought that the self-same ideals which you express color the life of 5,000 communities.

Great thinkers foresee a time when antagonistic laws and government divisions shall give place to one World Parliament. When that day comes, History will acknowledge the impulse to Peace resulting from the close relations established by commerce between nations. To that impulse you and your world-partners are daily giving greater force. The invisible bonds of sympathy which make of men whose names you may not know in the States, in Canada and in Mexico co-heirs of your great heritage have been flung across the waters. Today they interlink cities and hamlets in England, Scotland, Ireland, Wales, Hawaiian Islands, Cuba, Bermuda and the Philippines. The chain is endless; it encircles the earth.

Never before in all history have so many sources of individual power converged to one object. You belong to a brotherhood such as has been created by no human motive save religion since time began. That is suggestive. A spiritual element enters into every worldwide association of men, which preserves its existence. Without it there is no such thing as permanency. Turn the pages of the past, look abroad today, and you will realize the truth of this. Every great leader, however material his apparent purpose, succeeds in proportion to the degree in which his better nature finds expression in his work.

Remember that. And, when you figure profits, add to the material total the higher good which your heart knows is its truest reward. Rejoice when you prosper. For prosperity is the acid test of the age. But beware lest you pay the tribute which prosperity levies upon character. Financial success is the least important proof that you belong to the United Drug Company. Unless the fact shows in the clasp of your hand, in lifted head and level eyes; unless it is tacitly acknowledged by the instinctive turning of less fortunate men to you for sympathy, you are no true Rexallite.

Rexall Ad-Vantages continued for many years and it took on a digest form, but the nature of the contents never really varied—merchandising tips, success stories, some news, and plenty of ideas from Rexallites themselves. Indeed, for a time the magazine paid for ideas that were published.

Consumer Print Media

As noted earlier, Rexall published *Rexall News* for consumers. It was distributed through Rexall druggists and offered the opportunity to personalize each issue with the name of the individual drugstore. *The Rexall Magazine* followed with the same distribution plan, but with more stories, puzzles, and other entertainment interspersed, of course, with ads for Rexall products.

Sunday newspaper supplements, such as *Parade* and *This Week,* were regularly used for advertising Rexall products, as were national magazines. In 1950, for example, ads were to be found in *Life, Look, Saturday Evening Post, Collier's,* and *Country Gentleman.* Their combined circulation was sixty million.

Various other print media were also used, for example, *The Rexall Drug Store Family Almanac and Moon Book.* It was filled with arcane information, horoscopes, weather predictions, and, of course, Rexall ads. The 1950 edition featured actress Ann Blythe on the cover, and the first inside page reinforces the idea stated earlier that Rexall included the druggists themselves in its ads. It featured a generic picture of a druggist with the following message:

I'm your Rexall Druggist. In partnership with a great company I work to protect your health.

Working for you!

You've probably noticed that my store bears the Rexall sign. This means safe, sure, pure drugs for you. It means even more than that. That Rexall sign is a symbol of big business and little business working together to bring better drugs and better service to you and yours. Rexall gives you the very best in drugs and drug products. I bring you the skill required in compounding those drugs and add to it that personalized service which means so much. These two things—better drugs and better service—make Rexall a great name in your life. Look for our Rexall sign. Come in and see us. We're working together for you.

**You can depend on any drug product
that bears the name *Rexall***

The Golden Age of Radio

Radio offered a revolutionary opportunity for national advertising, and Rexall recognized this right away. The company produced its own shows, such as Rexall's *Parade of Stars* and *Rexall's Magic Hour* (home of the "Talking Penny"). Rexall sponsored such programs as *The Jimmy Durante Show* and the enormously popular *Amos 'n' Andy*. Certainly, the most interesting Rexall radio adventure was *The Phil Harris/Alice Faye Show* in the early 1950s.

The Phil Harris/Alice Faye Show:
The Rexall Family Druggist

The Phil Harris/Alice Faye Show is a special case for a number of reasons. It was sponsored by Rexall, and the company frequently figured into the story line, especially in the person of "Mr. Scott" (played by Gale Gordon), a mythical executive of the company. The show also featured a pharmacist, "Your Rexall Family Druggist," in a commercial role.

The use of the sponsor as part of the story was not a new device. Among others, Fibber McGee and Molly used the announcer, Harlow Wilcox, as a regular character whose recurring joke was finding a way to work a commercial message into a routine conversation. He did this with Pet Milk and Johnson's Wax, among others.

Phil Harris and Alice Faye played themselves, a band leader and singer/wife, with Rexall as their sponsor.[2] Ms. Faye was portrayed as having the brains and the money. Harris came off as vain about his looks (especially his curly hair) and not especially smart.

The show was a marvel of comic, slapstick timing. The writing was brilliant in the show and, in my opinion, in the commercials. The Rexall Family Druggist, played by Griff Barnett, delivered messages each show, many of which simultaneously informed and (presumably) sold, but also portrayed the pharmacist as knowledgeable and caring. The writers for the show were Ray Singer and Dick Chevillat.

Unfortunately, intensive inquiry among alumni of Batton, Barton, Durstine, and Osborne (BBDO), the advertising agency that handled the Rexall account, has failed to identify the author(s) of the commercials. These ads were a marvel of promotion in that they simultaneously sold the product and the credibility of the retailer (pharmacist) who delivered it to the customer. There has not been an equivalent performance in the drug industry since, which is why they receive such attention here. Bill Forman served as the announcer for more traditional (One-Cent Sale) commercials on the program.

Rexall in The Phil Harris/Alice Faye Show. Rexall was at least a "bit player" in all of the shows, but in some the company had a starring role. When that occurred the listener gained some insights into pharmacy and medicine. Always accompanied by laughs, these episodes presumably had an impact on listeners' views and opinions.

Ray Singer, one of the two primary writers on the show, explained that the writers had very little contact with the Rexall company. The audience, Singer believed, appreciated the fact that Rexall was a "good sport." The writers had one rule: "Never knock the product" (interview, March 23, 1988). Singer indicated that the script writers also had no contact with the advertising agency copywriters, and that there was no conscious effort to force the sponsor into the story line. If it was funny and natural to do so, they would, usually playing the Remley character off the sponsor. Singer, who has taught comedy writing at University of California at Los Angeles (UCLA), said that the students there still enjoy the humor.

Phil Harris, in an interview (March 4, 1988), indicated that he had little contact with Rexall, but that "integrated commercials" were part of the original "deal." Elliott Lewis concurred. Although he and Harris had one memorable meeting in the office of Justin Dart of Rexall, during which Dart played catch with a football in his enormous office, there was little exchange between the creative people and the commercial people (interview, March 21, 1988). Lewis noted that the practice of "working in" a commercial character allowed the sponsor to get around the very stringent rules on the amount of time that could be devoted to commercials. Some sample broadcast excerpts follow.

October 3, 1948: This was the first show with Rexall as a sponsor and the show revolves around the misadventures of Harris and Remley at Rexall Headquarters (including a drugstore). The stereotypes are introduced early. When Harris's daughters learn that he is going to work for "the biggest drugstore outfit in the country," they show their confidence: "You'll make the best sandwiches they ever had."

In this first show Remley introduces a line that is to be used as a recurring joke: "What's a Rexall?"

HARRIS: It happens to be one of the biggest drug companies in the world.

REMLEY: You mean that we are to be employed by a firm of apothecaries who manufacture pharmaceutical necessities?

HARRIS: Is that what they are? [With that information, Harris thinks he should get more money.]

March 5, 1950: In this program a member of the band asked Mr. Scott, "What's a Rexall?"

SCOTT: [*To himself*] They must be pulling my leg. They can't be that stupid.

HARRIS: They can too! Fellas, I'll explain what Rexall is. It's one of the world's foremost dispensers of "pharmaceutimanals." Furthermore . . .

SCOTT: That's enough, Harris. Their little minds are loused up enough without your explanation. I'll explain [*clears throat*]. A number of years ago a group of druggists formed a company. They needed a title to identify themselves, and after many months they came up with a grand old name. You know what they called it?

BAND: [*In disorder*] They called it Mary, Mary. [*Continue to sing*]

SCOTT: [*Outraged*] They didn't call it Mary. They called it Rexall.

BAND MEMBER: That's a silly name for a dame.

This willingness of Rexall to be the butt of jokes allowed the sponsor to be a part of the show. In some instances, Rexall was on the air for thirty minutes. It was fun, soft sell, and brilliant.

November 11, 1948: Surely the most fascinating show from a pharmaceutical viewpoint was this one, in which Phil Harris and Frank Remley decide to invent a new drug—using a children's chemistry set—to impress Rexall executives. Their logic is inescapable.

HARRIS: What makes you think they need a new drug?

REMLEY: Statistics.

HARRIS: He ain't even with the company.

REMLEY: Look, how many independent druggists have they got?

HARRIS: Ten thousand.

REMLEY: How many drug products do they make?

HARRIS: Two thousand.

REMLEY: All right. Ya see? That leaves eight thousand druggists without a drug.

The boys set to work, but first they need equipment, such as Bunsen burners. "You can't burn a Bunsen without 'em." The clerk in the scientific supply store is a bit reluctant to sell to anyone who is not a professional chemist, but they are quick to display their knowledge.

REMLEY: $H_2O_2O_2$ and carbontydioxide 5.

HARRIS: And if that ain't enough, Granite 3883.

The boys believe in serendipity, mixing chemicals at random and destroying a tablecloth in the process.

Moved by Alice to the garage, the boys find results in the Rexall colors, orange and blue, and need a "guinea pig." Julius Abbruzio is their candidate, but he will have none of it. In the struggle that follows, the test tube containing the new "drug" is dropped and explodes—to the benefit of all concerned.

September 25, 1949: Phil is assigned an office in the Rexall building and expected to keep regular office hours. He hates both. Mr. Scott (Gale Gordon), as head of Rexall, finds both Harris and his friend Remley incorrigible. He instructs Phil to think of something good for Rexall. Remley volunteers to help—"that ought to make the old pill-roller happy." The boys hit on a plan, in spite of their early failure in drug making.

REMLEY: What's one of the most beneficial drugs every discovered?

HARRIS: Penicillin?

REMLEY: Yeah. What do they make it out of?

HARRIS: Mold.

REMLEY: Okay. If mold is so good why don't we invent an aspirin made out of mold?

JULIUS: You think there'll be much demand for a moldy aspirin?

REMLEY: I'm talking about bread mold.

HARRIS: Bread mold? Common bread ain't good enough for us. Let's make it out of Rye Krisp mold.

REMLEY: Better yet. Let's make it out of seven-layer cake mold.

JULIUS: Why don't you make it out of Matzo mold?

HARRIS: Matzo mold?

JULIUS: Yes. Then your company will be the only one that sells Kosher aspirin.

Remley sees a remarkable opportunity for product line extensions—"Kosher Aspirin, Aspirin Cacciatore, Aspirin Stroganoff, Boiled Aspirin with Horseradish Sauce." (He would have found an exciting career in the 1970s as an OTC drug product manager.)

The boys give up on drug production and decide instead to run a One-Cent Sale. They do, selling *every* item for a penny. Harris is relieved of his office responsibilities.

The show closes with a serious message from Harris about the national polio epidemic.

December 5, 1948: In this episode, Frank Remley tries to fool his rich aunt into believing that he is married, settled, and successful. He "borrows" Phil's wife and children and introduces Phil as the man who does the radio program for the "Remley Drug Company." Remley's explanation of how "his" drug company has been converted to Rexall includes the note that he had to cut his product line from 50,000 to 2,000 products because he "couldn't find enough diseases to go around."

April 24, 1949: At the end of this show, Harris began a tribute: "Folks this is National Pharmacy Week . . . seven days when we can remember the man that you and your doctor trust all the year through, your family druggist. Quietly, but faithfully, these skilled professional men . . ." (At this point NBC interrupted, probably because time had run out.)

March 12, 1950: In this episode, Mr. Scott's daughter has a crush on Julius, giving Phil Harris serious concerns about his future with Rexall. This is a special problem, as Mr. Scott, the show's head man for Rexall, likes the young man, who in turn dislikes Harris.

The Rexall Family Druggist. One suspects that if you were to seek the word *avuncular* in the dictionary, you would find a picture of Griff Barnett as the Rexall Family Druggist. The commercials in which he talks to a radio audience or to "customers" in his drugstore are classics in promotion. The druggist comes across as kindly, but not obsequious; knowledgeable, but not paternalistic. Certainly, the sponsor's product benefits, but so, too, does the image of the retailer in the distribution channel. They impart knowledge, but knowledge that sells. With minimal changes they could (and should) be aired today. They would benefit the day-to-day industry of pharmacy. Several of them bear repeating here as examples of a (perhaps) lost art.

Most shows opened with some variant of the following message from the Rexall Family Druggist:

> Good evening. This is your Rexall Family Druggist taking a little time from behind the prescription counter with a welcome from the 10,000 independent druggists who have made the name Rexall part of our own store name. You can always tell us by the orange and blue Rexall sign in our windows. The sign means that we carry the 2,000 or more drug products made by the

Rexall Drug Company. They range all the way from aspirin to penicillin and they're as fine, and pure, and dependable as science can make them. [At this point a specific product was usually spotlighted—Milk of Magnesia, Bisma-Rex, Super Plenamins—but the last line was always the same.] You can depend on any drugstore product that bears the name Rexall.

Other introductory remarks by the Rexall Family Druggist (RFD) described such special events as the famous Rexall One-Cent Sale (cf. April 9, 1950). Sample transcripts follow:

RFD: Every once in a while we Rexall Family Druggists are asked this important question.

CUSTOMER: Why is a Rexall druggist different from any other?

RFD: Well, ma'am, the main difference is we were selected to carry the 2,000 or more products made by the Rexall Drug Company, and we take pride in recommending them to our customers.

CUSTOMER: They must be pretty fine products if druggists recommend them!

RFD: You hit the nail exactly on the head, ma'am. Let me give you an example of why we recommend them. Did you know, for instance, that drug products in tablet form should contain little or no moisture?

CUSTOMER: No, I didn't know that.

RFD: Well, it's true. And that's why, in Rexall's laboratories, there's a special apparatus that can detect as little as one one-thousandth of one percent of moisture. Before certain drug tablets are considered good enough to wear the Rexall label, they must meet their maximum moisture allowance as determined by this exacting machine.

CUSTOMER: Well, I'd say that's being pretty careful.

RFD: And I agree with you, ma'am. And we Rexall druggists know that all Rexall drug products get the same kind of painstaking, scientific testing and get it over and over again. That's why in every drugstore with the orange and blue Rexall sign in the window there's an independent druggist who will tell you, "You can depend on any drug product that bears the name Rexall." (January 9, 1949)

Another broadcast exhorted the wonders of Plenamines:

RFD: Last week a customer said to me . . .

CUSTOMER: I wish I knew some way to be sure I'm getting enough vitamins. Some way that's easy. Vitamins are expensive, too!

RFD: Ma'am, millions of people know how to do that. They take Plenamins, Rexall's popular multivitamin capsule. Plenamins cost only a few pennies a day and yet they give you more than your minimum daily requirement of every vitamin for which such requirements have been established. Plus, valuable liver concentrate and iron. And that's not me talking, ma'am. That's an iron-clad guarantee from Rexall scientists.

CUSTOMER: But just how are they able to guarantee that?

RFD: Because they measure the vitamin content of Plenamins with scientific accuracy. Take Vitamin C, for example. A Plenamins capsule is dissolved in solution and then a bluish dye is added in minute quantities and very, very slowly. The dye combines with the Vitamin C in the capsule and loses its color. Now this continues until the dye begins to overcome the Vitamin C and slightly color the solution. Thus, the amount of dye the solution has absorbed becomes an accurate measurement of the amount of Vitamin C in the capsule.

CUSTOMER: No wonder you Rexall Family Druggists sound so confident when you tell us . . .

RFD: You can depend on any product that bears the name Rexall? Well it's more than a slogan, it's a fact. (April 30, 1950)

In one program, the Rexall Family Druggist informs two female customers that every raw material used in a Rexall product has a case history:

RFD: . . . a complete record that tells what it is, where it's from, who made it and, most important of all, the results of all the chemical analyses made by Rexall's scientists. (November 28, 1948)

For one broadcast, aired at the height of the popular broadway show *South Pacific,* tickets were nearly impossible to obtain, so difficult that at the end of the show we find Rexall's Mr. Scott selling (so that he can see the show) "Peanuts, popcorn, hot buttered Plenamins." The real commercial follows, with a dissertation on tablet disintegration. When a customer is confused, believing the quality of Rexall aspirin lies in its ability to "dissolve real fast," the Rexall Family Druggist explains:

RFD: No ma'am. I mean they disintegrate real fast.

CUSTOMER: But what's the difference?

RFD: A great deal, ma'am. You see, aspirin itself is almost insoluble in water, and it's also too fine to hold together in tablet form. So, a way had to be found to bind it with an ingredient that would quickly disintegrate, that is, break up the tablet so the aspirin itself would immediately be free to do its job. (May 28, 1950)

He goes on to explain how Rexall scientists accomplished this by developing a "binder that begins to expand and come apart the minute it comes in contact with water."

Most of the Rexall Family Druggist's customers were female, but occasionally a man showed up with a question. In the February 5, 1950, commercial, for example, The Rexall Family Druggist explained to a male customer the use of the spectrophotometer to measure the amount of vitamin A in Super Plenamins.

A few months later in that same year, the subject was National First Aid Week:

RFD: Next week is National First Aid Week, seven days when the National Association of Retail Druggists calls your attention to the great need of proper first aid knowledge and first aid necessities that so often save lives. We are indeed proud tonight to salute the retail druggists of America as well as the 10,000 independent Rexall Family Druggists who are thus serving the communities and honor of this country. (May 14, 1950)

The only show in which any allusion is made to the identity of the Rexall Family Druggist aired on June 26, 1949. At the end of the episode, the druggist thanks the stars on behalf of the 10,000 independent druggists. Harris responds, "Thank you, Griff."

The Rexall Family Druggist was not exclusively occupied with explaining medications. On more than one occasion he was assigned to sell cosmetics. During the show on December 18, 1949, he informed the listeners that "we Rexall Family Druggists would like to play Santa Claus for all you tired last-minute Christmas shoppers." His suggestion was the Cara-Nome line of cosmetics for women and Stag for men. Both were Rexall exclusives. "We have Cara-Nome Cosmetics in delightful gift sets for as low as a dollar twenty-five up to a luxurious completely fitted travel case for seventy-nine dollars." The men's line had a much narrower price range—$0.75 to $15.95.

At the end of the December 25, 1949 Christmas show the Druggist spoke, not to his customers, but to other Rexall druggists:

> We're proud that you have chosen to make our family name part of your own. We're proud of the way the towns and communities you serve like and respect you, and of the active part you play in civic life. And so tonight, wherever you are, from Maine to California, from the St. Lawrence to the Rio Grande, Merry Christmas to you and to all your customers.[3]

In my opinion, the Rexall Family Druggist radio commercials were, for their purpose, among the finest ever produced. They enhanced the professional and human image of the druggist *and* provided compelling evidence that Rexall products were "as fine, and pure, and dependable as science can make them." As shown, typically they consisted of a conversation between the druggist and a customer, almost always female. In an unhurried and kindly fashion, the Rexall Family Druggist answered questions or volunteered information about Rexall products. Often the information he provided described practices used by the competition as well. *They* weren't on the radio, however, and it was easy to conclude that Rexall was the only drug company doing temperature testing, using special seals on their bottles, and so on—routine practices that were just unfamiliar to the public.

I have provided some verbatim examples, but much is lost in effect by being unable to hear them. You just had to trust this guy. I wonder how much the 10,000 or more Rexallites appreciated the value of these messages to them and their practices—and tried to capitalize on it.

As noted elsewhere, Rexall, in an economic move, dropped its sponsorship of the show, believing that the $14,500 cost per episode was too expensive. Even at that price it was still less than half that paid for the shows of Jack Benny or Bing Crosby. Perhaps Rexall didn't realize this particular bargain (*Alice Faye,* p. 200).

The Phil Harris/Alice Faye Show was not the only radio show sponsored by Rexall. *Amos 'n' Andy* followed immediately. In the May 1951 issue of *Rexall Ad-Vantages,* Rexall druggists were told the following:

> As this issue of your magazine goes to press, contracts are being drawn to wind up the final details and formal signing. Thus, the combination of "the best-known name in drugs" and the best-known comedy team in radio history will continue in partnership. And the show will continue to be aired over the entire facilities of the Columbia Broadcasting System.
>
> Never, since Rexall entered the field of big-time radio advertising, has your Company reached such massive audiences. More people have heard Rexall commercials each Sunday evening since January of this year than ever before. The fabulous comedy team has been consistently in third or fourth place among radio shows according to the Nielsen Ratings—a position never before held by a Rexall-sponsored network program.
>
> Equally astounding has been the flood of unsolicited and favorable comments from Rexallites everywhere. Without question, Rexall now possesses a radio program that has the enthusiastic approval of the entire Rexall family—plus an amazing record of support in Rexall store windows and on counters from coast to coast.
>
> Favorable public reaction began with the first show. The sincerity of the beloved team and the direct appeal of the commercial messages have been felt by Rexallites in every city and hamlet. A new customer who says, "Amos 'n' Andy asked me to drop in," has become a common occurrence everywhere.

This was followed by excerpts from letters received from Rexallites. The following two are typical:

Our first customer on Monday last called for Aspirin and wanted to make sure that they were "Rexall," and she said Amos 'n' Andy said to be sure to get "Rexall." Keep "shooting," we'll deliver the goods. . . .

A. J. PELOQUIN
H. L. FEARING
Centre Rexall Drugs
Southbridge, Massachusetts

On my swing through Kansas and Nebraska, I was dumbfounded to find the number of Rexallites who told me that one of their customers, or a person that might have been their customer, had come into the store and made the remark that Andy, of Amos 'n' Andy, had asked them to come in and get acquainted. . . .

L. R. YAGER
Rexall District Manager
Denver, Colorado

Frank Sternad has provided a delightful account of other Rexall-sponsored radio shows.[4] One was *Dan Carson's Story,* which was interesting in more than one way. The "hero" was "a Midwestern small-town Rexall druggist who typically becomes involved in the lives of his customers." (This is reminiscent of *County Seat,* a late 1930s' radio show starring Ray Collins [Lieutenant Tragg from *Perry Mason*] as a small-town druggist.) According to Sternad, and confirmed by him in an interview I was fortunate enough to have before his death, True Boardman, the writer/director/producer of the show, found ways, based on his own drugstore experiences, to incorporate "credible pharmaceutical dialogue into his scripts." Rexall products were mentioned by name during the stories and during the final episode. Phil Harris and Alice Faye visited Dan Carson's drugstore to plug their own show which was to follow in two weeks.

Besides sponsoring comedy/drama shows, Rexall provided other radio promotions for local use. In the 1951 *Rexall Ad-Vantages,* Rexall druggists were offered recorded radio commercials for use on local radio stations for their own sponsorship. The commercials were recorded by a professional announcer and featured musical signatures and a group singing "catchy Rexall jingles," including "Good

Health to all from Rexall." The cost per product, such as Puretest Aspirin, was only $2.50 per two-sided phonograph record.

Television Turns Up

Of course television would soon be added to Rexall's promotional bag of tricks. "Old time" radio was disappearing, to be replaced by the new medium. Rexall saw a chance to make the transition palatable. Here is a note from their 1957 annual report:

> Rexall's national advertising campaign reached a new high in impact on October 13 when, *for the first time,* an hour-long network television and radio "spectacular" was used to promote the Rexall One-Cent Sale. Spearheading Rexall's national advertising program, the NBC-TV and Radio simulcast of "Pinocchio" helped make this a record-breaking sale. The six-day event was the most successful One-Cent Sale in your Company's history.

> ### Pinocchio

> With an all-star cast headed by Mickey Rooney as "Pinocchio" and Walter Slezac as "Gepetto," this delightful musical adaptation of the ever-popular children's classic was hailed throughout the nation. Letters of praise and thanks poured in from viewers as well as Rexall druggists.

> Research data attest the show's widespread popularity. The A. C. Nielsen Company estimated Pinocchio's total audience at more than 50 million viewers. The Trendex rating service reported that over 50 percent of the sets in use were tuned to Rexall's Pinocchio.

> Rexall plans to launch its Spring 1958 One Cent Sale with a similarly delightful musical on Sunday, April 27. This time, it's . . .

> ### Hansel and Gretel

> Brought to you by the same production team who created and staged "Pinocchio," the "Hansel and Gretel" show is a lilting, light-hearted version of one of the world's best-loved fairy tales. Signed for starring roles are Red Buttons as "Hansel" and Barbara Cook as "Gretel," while Rudy Vallee and Risë Stevens will enact the roles of the Father and Mother. The "Witch" will be

played by Hans Conried and Stubby Kaye will be the "Town Crier."

Television differed from radio in many ways. Obviously, there was something to *see,* but it also tended to be too expensive to sponsor an entire program as had been the case with radio. Instead, short commercials (thirty or sixty seconds) became the rule on multisponsored television programs. Celebrities were often used as spokespersons (see picture section). According to the *Rexall Reporter* (1968), some 15,000 commercials were used in one campaign for the One-Cent Sale. They bought time on the big shows: *Today, Joey Bishop, Dating Game, Newlywed Game, The Tonight Show with Johnny Carson, Let's Make A Deal,* and others.

Miscellany

Super Plenamins ultimately became a real winner for Rexall, and one of the reasons was the way the product was tied into sports. In 1970 Terry Bradshaw was the National Football League's top draft choice and was signed to endorse the product. Rexall also contracted to sponsor the Olympic Games (1968) on radio from Mexico City. Super Plenamins and the One-Cent Sale shared airtime.

For a time, beginning in 1937, Rexall even advertised in medical journals: *Modern Medicine* and *American Journal of Medical Sciences.* As noted in Chapter 4, they featured Eudital, a "non-barbituric hypnotic." *Rexall Ad-Vantages* of February 1938 advised Rexallites of the ads and urged them to lay in a sufficient stock to fill the prescriptions that were sure to follow. The announcement described a twofold purpose—winning the goodwill of the profession for the Rexall stores (again remembering the Rexallites), and convincing physicians of the uniform high quality of United Drug pharmaceuticals.

CONCLUSION

It would be impossible to provide a complete chronicle of Rexall promotional activities over three-quarters of a century. Instead, I have tried to show Rexall's adaptability to available media, their resourcefulness and imagination, and the synergism that they tried to promote between the corporation and their 10,000 druggists—up until near the end.

PART III:
THE DART ERA

Chapter 8

Justin Dart:
A New Era of Genius

Justin Whitlock Dart is the second "larger than life" subject of this book. He was:

    a. A "boy wonder."
    b. A financial wizard.
    c. Ambitious and "let the devil take the hindmost."
    d. Easily distracted by opportunities.
    e. Other.

As in the case of Liggett, these and other possible sobriquets probably apply, depending on one's source of information (including the mass media and the time). One could include fascinating, flamboyant, and newsworthy under "e" above and surely be correct.

Dart was the sort of figure who attracts controversy. Opinions are divided on almost every issue concerning his role in the last three decades of Rexall history. Even the national media couldn't agree on who he was and what he stood for.

He made the cover of *Business Week* on July 13, 1946. In the accompanying article, the magazine noted that during his time at Walgreens, "It was his idea to clothe the chain drug store with flesh and blood by giving new dignity and emphasis to the prescription counter and the man behind it." Less than two weeks earlier (July 1, 1946), *Time* had reported that, at Rexall, "he buries prescription counters in the back of stores lest they take up valuable space for rag dolls, books, etc." Three years later, *Time* would describe him as an "aging Wonder Boy." *Time* didn't seem to like Dart very much. Perhaps they anticipated his role decades later in Reagan's "Kitchen

Cabinet," which was a major player both in Reagan's gubernatorial and presidential campaigns.

Let's take a look at how it all began.

DART'S EARLY CAREER

Dart was born in 1907 and played college football (tackle) at Northwestern University (all Big Ten). He was blessed with rugged good looks, plenty of personality, and strong merchandising ideas. He was hired after graduation as a stock clerk for the Walgreens organization by Charles R. Walgreen Sr., who, by all accounts, was greatly impressed by him and liked him personally. Also impressed, apparently, was Walgreen's daughter, whom Dart married. The marriage was a brief, childless one, and Dart later married a Hollywood "starlet," Jane Bryan. Apparently this did not affect his relationship with Mr. Walgreen, who, it is reported, remembered Dart very handsomely in his will (Rexall ms., p. 48).

DART AND UNITED DRUG

In 1941 Dart left Walgreens to join United Drug's Liggett chain as president. Two years later he became president of United Drug, replacing J. A. Galvin, who had succeeded Liggett upon the latter's retirement and now became chairman of the board. It is widely reported that Dart had been recruited by Montgomery Ward but chose United for a promise of broad autonomy. *Time* (July 1, 1946) confirmed an offer from Montgomery Ward but reported that Dart declined their offer of $150,000 a year in order to be allowed to move United to California and to continue at $75,000 per year. It didn't take long for him to exercise his new authority.

Early on, Dart focused on the drug business. (That would change later.) He had a vision of a chain of company-owned superstores (minimum of $250,000 annual volume and 4,000 square feet) and elimination of smaller, unprofitable company-owned stores—twenty-eight bit the dust in his first year.

In 1945 World War II was over, and Dart decided it was time to move. Choosing Los Angeles as the location for a new headquarters should have come as no surprise, even though a new headquarters remained to be built. The company had just purchased a converted B23 bomber that was used to transport books, legal records, and seals. It is reported (Rexall ms., p. 53) that the books were closed on Friday in Boston and reopened in Los Angeles on Monday.

Dart wasn't finished with his early changes. Under Liggett, United Drug had become a holding company for a variety of disparate companies. Dart began to bring order to the duplications and complexities that were a national part of such an "organization." He ordered the redesign of the packaging of all manufactured goods to feature the Rexall name. Then, with the concurrence of his board, he changed the name of the company to United-Rexall Drug Company, Inc. This change was supported by a national advertising campaign, including purchase of the rights to the *Jimmy Durante-Garry Moore Show* (Rexall ms., p. 54). In 1947 his firm became the Rexall Drug Company.

He didn't stop there. With 10,000 Rexall druggists to deal with, Dart felt that a modernization of the franchise contract was in order. The essence of the new contract was that dealers would be no longer compelled to follow any merchandising practice not enforced in the company-owned stores. In addition, more stringent rules were put in force regarding agents' participation in advertising expenditures and minimum purchase requirements.

As according to the old franchise, retailers also agreed to

1. participate in all major sales sponsored by United-Rexall Drug;
2. subscribe for, use, display, and pay for the monthly sales promotion service sold by United-Rexall Drug;
3. make use of United-Rexall Drug's monthly merchandising plans in formulating and carrying out his advertising and promotional activities;
4. devote at least 25 percent of all space used in their mixed merchandise advertising to United-Rexall Drug merchandise;
5. identify all their advertising as advertising of a Rexall drugstore;
6. use the advertising mat service distributed by United-Rexall Drug; and

7. share in the expense to United-Rexall Drug of any major advertising program sponsored by United-Rexall Drug for the purpose of promoting Rexall and the Rexall dealer or to promote
the sale of United-Rexall Drug merchandise. (This amounted to
0.5 percent of all Rexall purchases.) (Rexall ms., p. 54)

This revision of the franchise agreement seems to have been a
good move, at least according to *Time* (July 1, 1946), which reported
the following:

Independent druggists disliked the way the company sold them
its own manufactured products (candy, bandages, drugs, etc.)
with one hand and set-up competing chain stores with another.
Dart calmed the independents by closing off some of his weaker
competing chain stores and offering independents the benefit of
United's mass purchasing power. . . . United will now help finance the expansion programs of any affiliated druggists who
want to grow, hoping thus to build Dart's chain of super drug
stores.

Dart also planned to expand and diversify: "We'll buy plants in any
field where it would be cheaper to manufacture ourselves than to buy
on the market." History shows that Dart diversified far beyond this
limited plan.

In 1949 Dart threw a $90,000 party, with movie stars, searchlights,
and free orchids that was designed as an impressive kickoff to Dart's
postwar expansion plan. Unfortunately for Dart, the company was actually reporting a loss at the time, and he found himself firing some
2,500 of his staff, including some whom he had brought to California
(*Time,* November 14, 1949). Dart remained optimistic, however.

In 1950 Dart fought back. He experimented with a combination of
drugstores and supermarkets that would later become routine. According to *Business Week* (September 23, 1950), Dart's theory, pro-
ven to be correct, was that "housewives visit groceries four times as
often as drugstores. But once inside the grocery, they will be glad to
find a drugstore handy." Dart also provided a promotional innova-
tion—a packaged disc jockey program provided to the franchisees for
local use at a very low cost. According to *Business Week,* "For $4.50 a
program a small-town dealer gets a big-town radio show."

Nevertheless, times were tough in 1950. Rexall was losing money and economic cut backs were indicated. Some were rather curious. Facing a $1.25 million loss, *The Phil Harris/Alice Faye Show* became one of the victims of economic cuts. The show cost Rexall $14,500 a week, so Rexall substituted in its place *Richard Diamond, Private Detective* at $4,500 a week (*Business Week,* April 8, 1950). One can but hope that someone in the marketing department had a research-based notion that the decision was cost-effective, in other words, that the savings realized by this change were not negated by lessened sales from the advertising on the replacement show. We'll never know, of course, but the Harris/Faye show, because of its unique characteristics (see Chapter 7), *may* have been worth $10,000 more per week.

DART'S EXPANSION EFFORTS

In 1950 Dart took a major expansion step—still in the drug business—with Riker Laboratories, a first venture into prescription drugs. In 1952 Dart and Rexall acquired Vitamin Corporation of America, makers of Rybutol, one of the best selling-vitamin brands in the country—still in the drug business.

In the first half of the 1950s, Rexall continued slow but steady growth and divestiture of its company-owned retail stores, which, by 1955, numbered only 190, compared with nearly 560 just after World War II (*Business Week,* February 19, 1955). Shortly thereafter, Dart began his adventure in plastics. (And *The Graduate* wouldn't even be released until 1967!) This was a major departure from the product focus of Rexall. Although Liggett had diversified many times, every merger and acquisition was in some way related to the retail drug business. Certainly plastics, in the form of medicine vials and in other ways, could be seen as a part of the drug business, but Dart had grander ideas.

In 1958 Dart defied tradition by purchasing the Tupper Corporation and Tupperware Home Parties, Inc. *Business Week* (October 11, 1958) described the acquisition as "another step . . . in the campaign of Justin W. Dart to convert his company from primarily a retail drug chain to a major manufacturing enterprise."

Why did Dart change the central focus of his company? Many Rexall retirees felt that Dart never did plan a big future in retail drugstores; others felt that he grew bored with it. Dart himself answered the question regarding the deemphasis on retailing: "The profits are better [in manufacturing], and the long-range growth possibilities are better. In retailing about all you've got to look forward to is bigger overheads!" Such a statement should have sent shivers up the spines of Dart's 11,000 franchisees.

Tupperware was Dart's fourth venture into plastics. The first was the establishment of a Seamco Chemical division to manufacture, in plastic, products formerly made by its Seamless Rubber division. Next came Kraloy Plastic Pipe Company, maker of plastic pipes used in irrigation, oil fields, and chemical manufacture. This was followed by Chemtrol, as a tie-in to Kraloy. Dart was now a long way from the drug business.

Not that Dart was necessarily ignoring drugs. As noted earlier, his Riker subsidiary continued to develop new prescription drugs, and Dart expanded his drug and cosmetic manufacturing facilities in order to produce a new line of products for sale to non-Rexall outlets.

It should be pointed out here that during Liggett's fifty years prescription drugs were only a minor factor in drug retailing. The post–World War II era saw a boom in prescription drugs. These, with the exception of Riker products, had to be purchased from other companies, and any exclusiveness for Rexall stores was impossible. Surely Dart saw *something* written on the wall and was taking steps to adapt.

At this point Dart was not ignoring his franchisees. Indeed, as *Time* (August 18, 1958) reported, he "courted" them, inviting them to visit headquarters and have their pictures taken with Rexall executives for local newspaper publication, and providing attractively low wholesale prices on Rexall products. It was clear, however, that Dart was becoming disenchanted with the Rexall image as a drugstore company.

He told *Dun's Review* (April 1967), "This may sound strange coming from me, but it doesn't help Wall Street understand our company to have all those drug stores scattered about lower Manhattan." The magazine noted, "For Justin Dart to downgrade drugstores is a little like Dr. Land castigating cameras." Dart is quoted as telling visitors that his company is "not so much the Rexall *Drug* and Chemical Company as the Rexall Drug and *Chemical* Company"—*his* emphasis and obviously his view of the future.

By 1969 Dart's plans for the future were obvious when he announced the disposal of all of Rexall's drugstores, franchises, and proprietary drug operations, as well as the blue-and-orange signs and the Rexall name. The intended buyer was Commonwealth United Corporation.

In a letter to Rexallites, quoted in the 1969 first quarter issue of the *Rexall Reporter,* Rexall Drug Company President Robert Beattie (named president in 1968) tried to put a pretty face on the end of an era:

> The substantial initial investment by Commonwealth in our company, I believe, speaks well for the future and will give further impetus to the plans we have for building a stronger total franchise for Rexallites. Commonwealth United is a young, aggressive, growth-minded organization with substantial holdings in professional services, leisure products, oil, gas and entertainment.

Beattie's message continued with a look into the future and a realistic appraisal of things as he saw them:

> Today your company is a healthy, sound organization. It is important that you know this because only that kind of company can handle the products, the promotions and innovations that you need to run your business successfully. To me the future of the Rexall partnership is bright. Our product development program will produce a steady flow of high-volume products with which you can compete at retail and still make a good gross profit. We will continue to promote and advertise your store to make it more important in your shopping area. In short, we will do everything possible to make your Rexall franchise the most vital force in drug retailing and thereby your greatest business asset.

In fact, this sale, for reasons that are not known to this author, never happened. An article in *The Economist* (July 18, 1970) reported that Commonwealth couldn't raise the money. This was probably a confusing time, and a certainly confusing letter, for the franchisees.

Dart experienced some failures in his expansion efforts. His Vanda Beauty Counselors, an Avon "wannabe," never truly succeeded, but he never gave up, finishing his career with a merger with Kraft Foods to create Dart-Kraft in 1980.

Not everyone thought the union was a good one. Indeed, as reported in *Fortune* (July 14, 1980), one stock market analyst confessed, "I honestly haven't been able to figure out why Dart would want the deal." *Fortune* answers: "Why indeed? In large measure, the answer remains wrapped up in the ambitions of Justin Dart," a man who by this time had "purchased, created, or sold off upward of 50 different businesses." When concern was expressed about a possible loss of clout in the new organization, Dart was quick to reply, "I've always made my own clout." Nevertheless, when Dart died, his name disappeared from the company name.

As a footnote to the Dart saga, it should be noted that after moving to Los Angeles, in 1955, Dart handpicked John Bowles to serve as president of Rexall. By most accounts (see Chapter 3), it was an excellent choice. Bowles, according to his obituary in *The New York Times,* was the first to award a Rexall franchise to an African-American pharmacist. As noted earlier, he also brought a typical free-enterprise drugstore to the Poznan International Fair in Poland—a major coup in the cold war. Bowles died in 1993.

A FEW WORDS ABOUT WALGREENS

Walgreen deserves attention in a book about Rexall.[1] Walgreen was, after all, Justin Dart's alma mater, and he did marry Walgreen Sr.'s daughter, however briefly. Also, Walgreens provides an interesting parallel and contrast to Rexall in its history and later development.

Charles R. Walgreen Sr. and Louis Liggett could have been brothers. Each had a vision, and a seemingly inexhaustible store of ideas. In fact, Walgreen was a couple of years ahead of Liggett, and, unlike Liggett, he was a pharmacist. He opened his first drugstore in 1901 on the South Side of Chicago.

Walgreen is credited with the expansion of the soda fountain into a "luncheonette," thus becoming the cause of a thousand stereotypical jokes about druggists and grilled cheese sandwiches. One of his employees is credited with inventing the milkshake. Similar to Liggett, Walgreen immediately launched into private label products. The first, predictably, was his own ice cream. At the other end of the spectrum was his "Sure Death Bug Pizen" (for bedbugs). All of his products were guaranteed. Early on Walgreen, too, saw the advantage of strength in numbers and talked other neighborhood druggists into forming a co-op to pool purchases so as to exact lower prices from wholesalers.

Remember Liggett's trick of moving his staff around the plant to give the impression that there were more of them? Walgreen had a few tricks up his sleeve, too. He became famous for his "Two-Minute Start." Using new technology (the telephone!), Walgreen would receive an order, repeating each item very slowly and loudly so that his handyman could find and wrap the items. The handyman was quickly off to the customer's home (remember, it was a neighborhood drugstore) while Walgreen chatted amiably with the customer. Often that phone call was interrupted by the assistant's knock on the door, order in hand.

Walgreen is said to have been the first druggist to advertise on radio (more new technology). Similar to Liggett, he published a newsletter for customers, *The Pepper Pod,* which became very well known and lasted until the present. He named it to "reflect the stimulating nature of his growing enterprise" (p. 52).[2] Walgreens also played a major role in motion pictures, notably the film *My Sister Eileen* (1955). According to the company history, "Walgreens was one of the film's biggest stars" (*History of Walgreen,* p. 215). Bob Fosse, later a Tony Award and Academy Award winner, played the fountain manager in a Walgreens store. In a joint publicity campaign with Columbia Pictures, Walgreen supplied banners to his stores showing pictures of Fosse "mooning" over Janet Leigh as she sips a soda. The copy: "My Sister Eileen says . . . Walgreens is my favorite drugstore!"

By 1921 Walgreen had twenty-five stores and an empire was well on the way. Where Liggett had a train, Walgreen had a plane (see Chapter 7), which was flown to store openings over a period of four years (1937 through 1940). Some customers even won a free ride. By 1929 he had 397 stores. Walgreen encouraged employees to buy stock, as did Liggett, and his stock made the New York Stock Exchange in 1934.

Walgreen also established a Walgreen Agency system that was not unlike the Rexall franchise, with agents buying Walgreens merchandise and receiving promotional support. At one time, there were 4,000 agents, among them former Vice President Hubert Humphrey, a pharmacist himself, who worked in his father's Walgreen Agency in Huron, North Dakota. The agency system was discontinued in 1980.

Walgreens, too, supported the war effort, selling $41 million in war bonds and stamps. In the mid-1940s prescription volume was slipping, and this had always been an area of emphasis. (This was not a major focus for Liggett.) Chuck Walgreen Jr. was in charge now, and following consultation with the head of the American Medical Association, he directed his pharmacists to stop "counter prescribing"—essentially a practice of hearing patients' ills and selling them as over-the-counter products. Doctors didn't like that, and Walgreen told them when he stopped the practice. (This would seem incongruous to present-day "clinical" pharmacists.)

Walgreen took the brave step of initiating self-service in the 1950s, and, according to the company history (*100 Years,* p. 45), "by 1953 Walgreen's was the largest self-service organization in the country." In the 1960s, the company moved toward "supercenters," establishing seventeen by the end of the 1960s.

It should be noted that Justin Dart attempted the super drugstore with company-owned stores *and* provided financial incentives to franchisees who wanted to try expansion. It never worked out for him, and apparently he considered this a last ditch attempt at retailing.

In the 1950s, Walgreens took another innovative step that resembled the Rexall approach of training pharmacists and their trainers. Through an arrangement with the American Foundation for Pharmaceutical Education, Walgreens organized and presented an extensive seminar on the business of operating a modern drugstore. Faculty members from twelve colleges of pharmacy participated in the first seminar (*History of Walgreen,* p. 207). The seminars continued into the 1960s, "by which time virtually all colleges and universities were including a number of business courses in their pharmacy school curricula." (This is no longer true, but as a pharmacy administration professor for thirty-seven years, I personally have benefited from this Walgreens initiative.)

In the 1970s, Walgreen embraced the computer, and the company's computer network remains today one of its strongest marketing points. By the 1980s, Walgreens stores numbered more than 1,100, and by the year 2000 there were 3,000-plus. According to the company history, there is a target of 6,000 by 2010.

While Rexall was getting out of the retail drug business, Walgreens was getting stronger. We have seen many early similarities between the two companies (Walgreens even tried the One-Cent Sale), but there were important dissimilarities as well. The biggest was that Walgreens owned essentially all of its stores, whereas Rexall had 10,000 *independent* druggists. Financial incentives, assistance in merchandising, and all sorts of attempts at some coherence in marketing were used, but in fact it was the exclusivity of products that set it apart. Then, in a kind of desperation, they gave *that* away.

WALGREEN ON DART

The Walgreen Company–commissioned history (*History of Walgreen*) is not very kind to Justin Dart. Dart's behavior, described as "prankish," included the habit of firing a pistol into a stack of telephone books in his office (p. 154). On another occasion, he aimed a sand wedge he kept in his office at a box of talcum powder on the floor. With a practiced swing, he was able to cover an advertising salesman (and much of the office) in talcum.

Dart is described in *History of Walgreen* as taking credit for a number of successes for which he was not, in fact, responsible. His relationship with Charles Walgreen Jr. became strained for

- playing favorites with store managers;
- criticizing Walgreen's conservatism and suggesting that he, Dart, would have made a better president;
- attempting to have repealed a state law requiring that the president be a pharmacist (Walgreen was; Dart was not); and
- failing to consult with board members on important policy matters.

Although he was not without his supporters, Dart was described as believing himself to be a "one-man team," not a team player. In July 1941, the board unanimously called for his resignation. True to form, Dart asked for (and received) permission to use the company plane to seek another position. He found one—with Rexall.

CONCLUSION

This chapter was about Justin Dart. Some say he grew bored with the retail drug business, some say he gave up, and some say he got big stars in his eyes. It is difficult to find anyone who will assert that Dart simply faced the fact that the old Rexall model wouldn't work in the face of competition with modern drug chains, Wal-Mart, Kroger, and the like, not if he wasn't able to control his once powerful retail empire—and control was what had led him to come to and stay with United Drug in the first place.

Some would accuse Dart of being less than gracious in his remarks about Liggett, as reported in the September 15, 1967, issue of *Forbes* (well after Liggett's death). He did give Liggett credit for a great idea, "for its time," but criticized his handling of the Boots purchase and sale. With characteristic "humility," Dart said, "It was anything but a sound company when I joined in 1943."

Chapter 9

The End of the Rexall Era

Here's how the end of Rexall, as we knew it, seems to have come about. First, as already noted, Justin Dart had a larger vision than simply being CEO of "that drug company." Mergers and acquisitions came thick and fast. Diversification was not foreign to the company Liggett had founded. Merwin (*RFA*, p. 142) said of Liggett:

> He meant to come pretty close to manufacturing every imaginable item that could reasonably be sold in a drug store; and the only way to do that was to own the factories that made them—note paper and envelopes, rubber goods, cotton factories, glassware, pure foods, and preserves, prescription drugs as well as the proprietary remedies, sugar, toilet articles, soda fountain supplies, candies of all sorts, veterinary medicines and remedies for dogs, cats, horses and cattle—just about everything!

Dart, in contrast, seemed more interested in acquisitions—any acquisition, not just those designed to stock the drugstores of his Rexall franchisees. This was obvious, in part by the company name change, in 1969, from the Rexall Drug and Chemical Company to Dart Industries.

An early company directory for Dart Industries listed the following companies:

Action	Colorite
American Gasket	Consolidated Thermoplastics
Aztec	Coppercraft
Babcock Phillips	Dart Resorts
Canada Cup	Electrochemicals
Capital Controls	Environmental Research
Century Fiberglass	Fiberfil

Fluid-Ionic Systems
Heil
Imco
Lancy
Nappe-Smith
Nissin-Dart
Plastic Clad
PureChem
Ralph Wilson Plastics
Rexall
Rexcel
Rexene Polyolefins
Rexene Styrenics
Rexpak
Seamco
Seamless Hospital

S.E.P.
Southwest Latex
Styro Products Europe
Synthetic Products
Syroco
Thatcher Glass
Thatcher Plastics
Thermo-Serv
Thompson
Tupperware
Vanda Beauty Counselor
Weden Tool
West Bend
Wilson Products
Woodtape

Rexall was now just one of forty-five companies in this patchwork conglomerate that included plastics, gaskets, and resorts. Dart would later enter into a merger with Kraft Foods, as reported in Chapter 8.

Dart went shopping for a buyer for Rexall. (With his holdings, why not buy one of his companies and get another for a penny?) His first buyer was the Commonwealth Company of California. That 1969 deal fell through, but in 1977 Rexall was sold to a group of investors from Dallas known as Ross-Hall for a reported $16 million. A holding company, Ross-Hall had no experience in the drug business. Some have the opinion that the Rexall acquisition was planned as a tax writeoff.

At this point, the unraveling of the original Rexall concept was completed. The decline in commitment to the original Rexall concept had begun earlier. Rexall was doing okay in the late 1950s—indeed, profits tripled in 1959 from the previous year—but things were being changed. The 1961 annual report noted, "Rexall Drug Company's program of extending franchises to selected retailers *continued* in 1961. The largest new franchise signed during the year was by Crown Drug Company, a thirty-seven-store chain in Kansas City." Wait a minute! Weren't the chains the nemesis of the independent? What about the existing franchisees in Kansas City?

Change didn't stop there. Rexall products were now sold through wholesalers and even to other retailers at large. No wonder franchisees would become disenchanted with their relationship with Rexall. After the Ross-Hall takeover, changes were both dramatic and obvious. In 1979 Rexall President Howard Vander Linden described plans for the future in the first issue of *Rexall Review,* an employee publication:

1978 was a building year for us in which we continued to sacrifice operating profit by holding down prices in order to gain distribution in the marketplace. With the continuing promotional emphasis on nutritional products, 1300 more retail outlets are now handling Rexall vitamins and other products than did at the first of the year. Major chains such as Skaggs (St. Louis, Memphis and Phoenix); Medi Mart (Boston); Gray (Cleveland), and Genovese (New York) are all now featuring Rexall vitamin products.

One of the most significant changes in marketing direction occurred in 1978 with the startup of the Rexall College Vitamin Program. 110 of America's leading colleges and universities now handle Rexall vitamins in their book stores, introducing young people who will be returning to their communities, we hope, confirmed Rexall vitamin users. Harvard, Yale, Missouri, U.C.L.A., Alabama, Minnesota, Brigham Young, Texas A&M, Washington, Princeton, plus a hundred more, sell Super Plenamins and other Rexall vitamins.

In 1979, we will be widening Rexall distribution further afield with the help of a new advertising agency. Plans are now being formulated to take several key Rexall brand products on a "national" distribution basis. We will first be test marketing and advertising in metropolitan areas key brand-name products including Super Plenamins; and then later in 1979, roll out into major geographical sections of the country into drug, food and discount stores backed with heavy advertising.

1979 will see a further reduction of non-manufactured products and a substantial increase in the promotion of factory-produced products. As time goes on, Rexall will become known more as a manufacturing/marketing company and less as a drugstore-oriented retailer.

In 1980 Larry Weber took over as president of Rexall and initiated a cataclysmic change: He simply canceled the contracts with the 10,000 Rexall druggists. Weber, quoted extensively in a March 1, 1982, article in *Business Week,* explained "We're much more than just a drugstore now," he said. "We're mass merchandisers. Where we could only reach 10,000 stores in the past, our products can now reach 200,000 stores. I feel like Colgate-Palmolive and Procter and Gamble." That would never happen, of course, and Liggett must have been spinning in his grave. Weber changed Rexall from primarily a manufacturer to a distributor. He cut the company workforce by a third, and the remaining sales force was especially hard hit.

The *Business Week* article quotes one Rexall executive as saying: "[Weber] decimated the place, destroying employee morale." The sales force that remained after the cuts was, according to another quoted executive, "unprepared to market to one-time [Rexall] retail competitors." The executive continued, "The company is too dependent on a sales force that catered to its own mom and pop stores and not to the sophisticated retail chains that increasingly dominate the industry." Surely Rexall franchisees would take issue with the "mom and pop" label. At one time that might have been near the truth, but in the 1980s most were significant retail outlets. Besides the pejorative term seemingly in use at Rexall headquarters, the franchisees (thousands of them) could hardly be expected to welcome the Rexall salesperson, having been recently abandoned by Rexall.

The *Business Week* article continued with a description of the fate of Rexall drugstore signs, further evidence of Rexall's ambivalence:

> There are still thousands of drugstores that wear the Rexall name. They are former franchisees who have been permitted to use the logo because Weber wants more visibility for the Rexall brand name. Whether that is a good idea is also questionable. Many Rexall outlets were small, old stores that one former executive describes as "eyesores." Some of them undoubtedly are conveying a negative public image.

Weber's dreams did not come true, and he was replaced (or resigned) as Rexall's president. Manufacturing problems in St. Louis caused a loss of confidence by customers, and a plan to remodel and modernize the St. Louis facility never materialized. Debt increased and the major lender refused to provide more capital. According to Taylor (*Rexall Story,* p. 41), the Rexall assets were sold to a Florida organization called the Rexall Group in 1985. Then, in 1989, the Rexall name was purchased (for something between $35,000 and $75,000) by the Florida-based Sundown company. It seems somehow appropriate, but also sad, that the sunset of Rexall should occur with its sale to Sundown.

Chapter 10

Conclusion

Was Louis Liggett a man (genius) of his times? We have seen how he attempted to create an organization of retail druggists through providing exclusivity for sale of the Rexall line of nonprescription drugs and other drugstore products. Prescriptions received very little attention in his scheme of things. Why was that so?

For one thing, Liggett was not a pharmacist, but rather the ultimate merchandiser. His approach to Rexall is best summed up in his own words concerning pharmacists and their drugstores. I believe the extensive quotation that follows is warranted for the insight it provides into Liggett's views. It comes from a series of three articles written by Liggett in the February, March, and April issues of *The Pharmaceutical Era* in 1914. The series was titled "Pharmacy in the Past Twenty-Five Years" and published ten years after Liggett began his retail adventure.

Professional Ideals.

The druggist of 25 years ago called himself an apothecary and considered himself a member of one of the learned professions. He believed that there was a difference between pharmacists and business men, and that the difference was in his favor. In his regard for professional ethics he paid little heed to the larger ethics of public service. He never put it into words, perhaps, but he thought that dignity and small net profits were somehow related. He was certainly not a merchant. He sold toilet goods, perfumery, brushes, etc., but he did not feature them. The goods were shown when asked for, and when sold yielded the same ratio of gross profit as was charged for drugs, which was always double and sometimes more.

The Old Store.

I remember as though it were yesterday, the typical old-time drug store. In its windows were jars of colored water which served a purpose by calling attention to the store when electric signs were unknown. Also, there were festoons of dusty sponges, exhibits of cochineal bugs, rock sulphur, and fly specked cards announcing the "Old Folks' Supper" at the Methodist Church.

Profitable Goods Not Shown.

But it was inside the store that the difference between the old druggist and the new was most evident. In the old store the front shelves, which are now devoted to attractive goods selling themselves to well people—candy, stationery, perfumes, etc.—were filled with glass-labeled jars and tincture bottles. The fact that the sight of Syrup of Squills or Tr. Asafetida never stimulated the buying instinct did not worry the professional pharmacist, any more than did the fact that by keeping the tinctures in the front of the store, he was forced to make unnecessary trips back and forth to the prescription case. . . .

Commercial Standing.

Though always respected for his high integrity, the old-fashioned druggist did not enjoy a very high commercial standing in his community. Owing to his semi professional character he was more likely to be asked to contribute to local campaigns than to take active leadership as he does today.

Location of Stores.

The retail druggist has always been fortunate in the matter of location. Twenty-five years ago, as now, the most prominent corner in the town was almost invariably occupied by the druggist. One might almost say that the best corner was tacitly reserved for him. The drug store of early days was quite as prominent as the store of today. For while the modern druggist has electric signs, "flashers," beautiful store fronts and striking color-schemes with which to draw attention, his predecessor got something of the same results by using the familiar colored window bottles, which, with the light shining through them, beaconed trade and were the most brilliant illuminations on the street. . . .

The Pharmacist Compared with Other Retailers.

The question is often asked: "How did the early pharmacist compare with other retail business men?" The answer is that there was no comparison. For, as said before, the pharmacist was a professional man and was not considered when merchants were thought of. . . .

The Prescription Department.

The general feeling among druggists is that the prescription department is very profitable. My knowledge, based upon figures, is that it is not such a profitable department, and has not been profitable for the past 10 years. In fact, each year it becomes less and less profitable, not necessarily in all stores, but in the average stores throughout the United States.

There was a time when 60 percent to 65 percent gross profit could be made in the prescription business. Today it is very difficult to get 45 percent, owing to the fact that many prescriptions are written for nothing more than such established proprietary articles, as Gude's Peptomangan, Fairchild's Essence of Pepsine, etc. *The day of compounding has gone by,* and it was compounding that made the prescription department profitable. Those retail druggists who have kept prescription costs tell me that there is very little left in the prescription business, and yet it is a department, which, if properly conducted, requires a heavy investment.

Old Druggist Passing.

And now, what is the ultimate effect of this diversification of the retail druggists' business? Is the purely prescription pharmacy extinct or soon to become so? The question—Could a druggist confining himself to a prescription business remain in existence today?—is sufficiently answered by the experiment conducted in New York a few years ago. A purely prescription pharmacy was opened at that time, and though a very large business was transacted it proved unprofitable without the side lines, which are the main source of income in the merchandising store.

Has the so-called ethical druggist passed into oblivion? To this question I think the answer is affirmative, and it is unwise to harbor vain regrets. In a retrospect of the past 25 years I can see many characteristics, many elements that I would, were it possible, incorporate in the modern retail drug store. For the pioneers in this business were splendid workers, men of real nobility, who thought the sacrifice of time and money and all that made life worth living, a small price to pay, if thereby they could maintain their profession at the level of their ideals. They won public confidence by the integrity of their character and their fair dealing. They have left that confidence to us as our heritage.

While I glory in the wonderful progress that is being made by the drug merchants of today; while I believe that the drug business is on an ascending arc of evolution; while I see ultimate good, even in those tendencies which others deplore, yet I am firmly convinced that the real success of the drug business depends not upon departmentizing, the solving of the overhead problem, frequent turnovers, advertising and all the rest of it, so much as it depends upon the extent to which we prove worthy of our heritage, and whether or not we give it into the hands of our successors unsullied.

Liggett seems to have been somewhat ambiguous in his views of the prescription department. Merwin (*RFA,* pp. 90-91) reported that one of Liggett's

> earliest steps in expansion (a modest one) was to supply material for prescription work—the standard drugs of the pharmacopoeia. They were equipped to do it. Furthermore, many drugs cannot be kept long and will deteriorate in quality on the shelves of the druggists' back room. He could organize a system of frequently supplying fresh material. A real service, this. So he laid his proposal before the Board of Directors, on an occasion which one of them recalls amusingly. Already Liggett had proved himself many kinds of man. He hadn't stumbled yet, at any point. But he was no pharmacist. Not then. With the aid and advice of experts he had prepared a long list of the prescription drugs he proposed to manufacture and distribute. Painstakingly he read it off. The difficulty was that most of the names were long and alien. He couldn't pronounce them at all. The directors laughed. He himself laughed. They saved the situation by simply authorizing him to go ahead. He was always going ahead anyway, so they might as well. He'd be a master of the subject before long. He is now a Doctor of Pharmacy, with a diploma from the Rhode Island College of Pharmacy.

"The day of compounding has gone by," wrote Liggett. How much truth was there in this, and, if even only to a large extent, what were the reasons? An extensive explanation for the decline in the number of prescriptions was presented by M. S. Kahn at a meeting of the Baltimore Retail Druggist's Association in June 1913, the year before the Liggett series. It was also published in *The Pharmaceutical Era.* I hope the reader will accept a necessary long quotation:

> The surgeon, the X-ray, radium, and what not, have all helped to diminish the number of prescriptions, but I really think the more truthful part is expressed by Dr. Henry Beates, president of the Pennsylvania State Medical Examining Board, at a recent meeting of the Philadelphia branch, A.Ph.A., giving an answer to the question, if there is a crisis in the drug trade, which would have raised a storm of protest if it had come from a druggist. Dr. Beates plainly said that the reason why the druggist does not receive more prescriptions for galenical preparations is that physicians did not know how to formulate a prescription of the proper drugs in the proper combination best suited to the patient or the conditions of the case. Furthermore, he asserted that few of the present-day practitioners know the exact therapeutic action of drugs; that not one in ten could tell the difference in the effect produced by an infusion of digitalis made from a fluid extract and that produced by one made from the assayed leaf, giving this as an example of the lamentable lack in the study of materia medica and in positive knowledge of drugs.
>
> One of the chief causes assigned for the decline in the prescribing of preparations, the dispensing of which requires skill and learning on the part of the druggist, therefore, was the insufficient teaching of materia medica in medical colleges, the subject usually being given in the first year and promptly forgotten in the succeeding years when all of the student's time is taken up with the refinements of diagnosis, pathology, bacteriology and other modern additions to the curriculum. The graduate, it was said, could diagnose a case in the most exact manner, but when he came to prescribe the proper drug or combination of drugs for it, he was all at sea and in despair, would prescribe something made by somebody which he remembered to have been told was the exact remedy required. And the worst part is the fact that the prescriber not only does not know what he is prescribing, but does not even know how the remedy ordered acts upon the patient, except that he gets better or worse.

It is a fact, as any druggist knows who has watched the prescription file dwindle, that physicians are prescribing less and less carefully thought-out combinations of drugs and pharmaceutical preparations and are relying more and more on ready-made combinations. Here is the opportunity for the druggist to prove his worth as the real assistant of the physician. Let him show the medical man that he has not only the knowledge to select and the skill to prepare the best preparations of each drug, but that he also knows something of its therapeutic action. This does not mean that we should try to instruct the physician, for such attempts would be resented, but that he should keep informed by raiding both pharmaceutical and medical journals, and should have a file of these and of the latest authoritative books on materia medica. There are not enough prescriptions written now to go around, so the druggist who wants a prescription business must build it up by showing physicians not only his qualifications for compounding but also his ability to help them over difficulties arising from their lack of knowledge of materia medica and the therapeutic efficiency of drugs. Tact and unassuming helpfulness will overcome the distrust that now exists on the part of physicians.

This was the situation in which independent druggists found themselves in the early part of the twentieth century. Some retail druggists—Squibb, Lilly—turned to manufacturing; most could not.

Post–World War II the situation changed. The pharmacist's compounding function had been usurped by drug manufacturers and was manifested by an explosion of prefabricated prescription remedies. Here was a chance for the independent druggist to recapture the prescription business. But as the second half of the twentieth century—the Dart Era—evolved, so did the chain drug industry.

Walgreens is a good example of how a chain could exploit professional service and the lower prices made possible by their purchasing power. The price-cutting that could be combated by Rexall's exclusive store brands was not possible with prescription drugs. It wasn't long before grocery store chains, variety store chains, and superstore chains were in the prescription arena, after using the prescription department as a loss leader.

So did the independent druggist whose future was filled with promise by Rexall disappear? No, but Rexall did. Thousands of independent druggists have found specialty practices, niche locations, and professional services that patients value as much as a discount, but they aren't Rexall. Whether Dart and colleagues were smart enough to see these developments in advance or simply adapted and reacted as change occurred really doesn't matter. What *does* matter is that *perhaps* a proper commitment to helping their franchisees adapt and react *may* have saved Rexall. It didn't happen and perhaps never could have.

Afterword

I know now that I began this project with a number of biases. Having grown up, literally and figuratively, in the era of the "independent druggist," I felt that a tremendous opportunity to save that retailer must have been lost when Rexall ceased to exist. Probably my vision was partially obscured by a pharmacy teaching career in Mississippi. Certainly most of my practicing pharmacist colleagues were drugstore owners. Chains were slower to come to our state than to many others, and there was a kind of insularity—even though I claim to be widely read and widely traveled.

Changes that *I* knew about but did not initially bring to this project were internal to the profession of pharmacy. Among the major changes were the following:

- As the century proceeded, new recruits from pharmacy families, especially independent pharmacy families, became fewer and fewer.
- As chains grew in number and influence, high school students had access to fewer drugstore owners as role models.
- There was a dramatic increase in the proportion of female students. For a variety of reasons, women seemed to be far less likely to be interested in owning a drugstore.
- New, exciting opportunities emerged in various institutional and clinical pharmacy practices.
- Courses in pharmacy management and merchandising virtually disappeared from pharmacy curricula.
- The money for chain practice became very attractive, especially to students burdened with loans.

There were other factors, of course, but the fact is that the raw material of Rexall, the pharmacist committed to entrepreneurship via independent pharmacy ownership, was simply drying up. Too bad.

Appendix

A Profile of Hazard Rexall Drugs

AN INTERVIEW WITH JOE DUNCAN, OWNER, HAZARD (KENTUCKY) REXALL DRUGS, 1952-1989

This interview is included for the personal insight it provides into the relationship between Rexall and their franchisees. After nearly forty years as "Rexallites," the Duncans are well qualified to comment. I appreciate their help and cooperation. The interview has been edited for the sake of continuity.

SMITH: I have jotted down a few questions, and I'd just like to run through them. Where did you get your pharmacy training?

MR. DUNCAN: Where did I go to school? It was the old Louisville College of Pharmacy, and it's no longer in business.

S: I'm aware of it.

MR. D: I went just after the University of Kentucky had taken it over, but it was still the same faculty and the same building, but my degree says "UK."

S: What year did you finish with that?

MR. D: My degree says 1952.

S: You got your store in 1959. Is that right?

MR. D: No, I got the store in 1952.

S: Boy, you did better than I did. I thought I was going to get a drugstore when I graduated, but I didn't make it.

MR. D: It was too much, through trials and tribulations, but we got it off the ground.

S: Was it a new store?

MR. D: No, it was one that had been in existence since 1912.

S: Boy, oh boy, that really did have a rich history, didn't it? Was it a Rexall store then?

MR. D: Always was, as long as Rexall *was*.

S: So you bought a Rexall store and you stayed with Rexall as long as they lasted. Right?

MR. D: As long as they lasted.

S: How was your relationship with Rexall and their salespeople, etc.?

MR. D: You mean with Rexall? Basically good until near the end. When they came up with the new franchise, a bunch of us Rexallites got together at Danville, and this one boy got up and said, "You know what that franchise says? It says that you can run a Rexall store in your building. And that's it. Somebody could put one in right next door if they wanted to."

S: They messed it up really bad at the end.

MR. D: Yes, when they changed over . . . Justin Dart, etc.

S: Well, they sold it to a group called Ross-Hall, so far as I can tell, and they are the ones who really blew it. What were the best things Rexall did for you?

MR. D: Well, I'll put it this way. Everybody knew our store as Hazard Rexall Drug Store, but everybody just said Rexall. Of course, the profit markup was good on everything. It was very satisfactory.

S: That's what I keep hearing. Tell me about the end, when things started going bad.

MR. D: I really don't remember. What year did they go out?

S: I think they sold out in 1977. I know they started selling some of the stuff through wholesalers and to other stores. I think Plenamins was the big one. One of my hobbies is old-time radio. I have a bunch of tapes. Do you remember *The Phil Harris/Alice Faye Show* and the ads?

MR. D: I remember the ad we had on the radio that said something about "Good health to all from Rexall. We hope you are doing fine."

S: For a couple of years they sponsored a show called *The Phil Harris/Alice Faye Show.*

MR. D: I don't remember it.

S: I wish you did, because at the end of it, there was a fellow who called himself the Rexall Family Druggist and he talked about all the good things Rexall was doing and that Rexall druggists were doing.

MR. D: What year was that?

S: I think this was 1952 or 1953.

Mr. D: I was just starting out then.

S: You told me the other day about the One-Cent Sale. I know that was a major thing every year.

MR. D: We preordered for that. We even had advance order forms where people could pick them up, fill them out. We had a lot of fun with it. I remember one thing that isn't of any major importance. You have been in a store, and you recognize these tightwads that won't buy anything unless it is a real big deal. Well, on the sale paper it had safety pins in plastic containers, one big one and ten or twelve in descending size. This one man and his wife had filled out this form and they had put down to get two of them. He came back in about thirty minutes, and he said, "This isn't what it says on the paper I'm supposed to get. It says I'm supposed to get two of these big canisters." I said, "No, I'm afraid not. . . . I'll just give you the eleven cents back."

S: One of my friends down here who was in a Rexall drugstore said there were some people they only saw twice a year.

MR. D: Yeah, well they'd buy your Klenzo and Mi31. And I swear to God I couldn't believe the glycerin suppositories we used to sell.

S: You wouldn't think there would be that big a market for them.

MR. D: I couldn't believe there would be that many people who used glycerin suppositories.

S: Just to save some money.

MR. D: They would get eight or ten at a time.

S: I had a picture here in Oxford, and on the day of the sale, you couldn't get around the drugstore—they had so many cartons and stuff in it.

MR. D: We didn't have room to do that out front. We had it all inside.

S: What did you feel like when Rexall started coming apart?

MR. D: Well, kind of like you have been sold out.

S: That's what I have been hearing.

MR. D: Yeah, I really hated it.

S: Did you keep your store?

MR. D: Yeah, I kept the store. I closed it in 1989, because our downtown took the route of so many downtowns when the Wal-Marts and Kmarts and so forth came in.

S: That's the way it is here. There's still one drugstore downtown, but they don't do anything. Did you keep the sign?

MR. D: Yeah, the sign was up there, but I sold my fountain equipment and all that to a fellow who put in a little sandwich shop, and he just painted over that sign and it said "Hazard Sandwich Shop," I think. They couldn't fuss about that. The building has burned down since then, so all of that is gone.

S: That's what I understood from your Web site . . . that you had a fire, and that's a shame. Did you get some kind of notice from Rexall saying, okay, the franchise thing is over?

MR. D: Yeah, something to that effect. I don't remember the exact wording, but it was to that effect.

S: If you have anything there at home, like old forms or pictures of the store when you first started or any of that kind of stuff, I have got quite a bit of material that I am going to be using in the book. I will make the copies down here and get them back to you in good shape.

MR. D: I thought I had somewhere one of those plaques on a wooden stand honoring us for being good Rexallites.

S: I saw one somewhere that had the Aesclepius on it. I don't know what the purpose of that one was. But he let me take that one home with me.

MR. D: Here, Elizabeth will describe this thing to you.

MRS. D: It has a mortar and pestle on top and some sort of design on the side . . . lions or something. The plaque is awarded to Hazard Rexall Drug by the Rexall Drug Company for outstanding achievement. Here's the president's name . . . John Bowles. It was in 1957.

S: He was hired by Justin Dart.

MR. D: Well, that's about all I've got. It was nice talking to you.

The Hazard, Kentucky, Web site (hazardkentucky.com) contains comments from former customers and employees. Perhaps they provide the best possible reflection on a part of Americana that, according to the Web site, now exists in cyberspace.

> I read my first comic book from the rack stand at Rexall Drug and had my first banana split there also. After Sunday School and Church on Sundays always had to have a cherry coke. Thanks for the memories! (Angelene Boyas North, Bradenton, Florida)

> My last visit to Hazard was in July 1987. I worked at the Hazard Rexall Drug from 1960 through 1962 at the soda fountain. I worked for Joe Duncan. He was a very nice person to work for. One of the ladies who worked with me was named Avonelle. I am so sorry to know that with my next visit, I will not be able to visit Rexall Drug. (Clara Davidson Nordstedt, Gainesville, Florida)

> I was born and raised at Hardburly. I remember the drugstore and visited often. My wife of forty-five years worked there when she was in high school. In later years we would stop in when we came home to visit. Claudia passed away in September 2000. With the loss of the drugstore and Claudia my world became smaller. (Chester Lawson, Troy, North Carolina)

> I remember going over to Hazard Drug for a PayDay and a Pepsi. Every now and then I would get a lemonade. It never tasted the same

anywhere else. Also, the pimento cheese sandwiches. (Joe Eversole, New York, New York)

I was a teenager in the late 1940s working there. It was a fun place to work; everyone knew everyone in town. Our city policeman came in every day for refreshments and to give us a hard time. One of them was a real stinker, soooooo to get even with him we put SAL-A-PATIKA in his milkshake. Well that kept him home for a couple of days. I often think of my hometown and hope to go back some day. Thank you for this Web site. I have been able to keep in touch with my dear friends from the past. I was able to locate one friend I had lost track of after fifty years. Keep up the good work. (Betty Strong Hobbs, Fort Wayne, Indiana)

I worked at the Hazard Drug. I'm so sorry to hear that it burned. Gosh it's been fifty-plus years ago that I worked there, but I can never forget all of the sodas, sundaes, and milkshakes I made and the coffee I poured. I also made some lasting friendships there. I remember the Hazard Drug as a fun place to work, I sure wish I could have seen it once more and enjoyed a cup of coffee or a soda at the fountain. I live in Texas now and haven't been back since 1983. I have so many fond memories of Hazard and all the places I worked, and all the nice people there. (Vera Feltner Hudson)

One thing I liked about Main Street was every morning about ten o'clock everybody that had a business on Main Street used to slip out the back door and go down to Hazard Drug because they charged a nickel for a cup of coffee. The other places charged a dime. We'd go in there and have a meeting and straighten out the world situation and have a cup of coffee and swap a few tall tales. (Hazard Photographer, Hal Cooner)

I'd window-shop all the way to the parking lot at the east end of Main Street, stopping in Rexall Drugs to look at and buy comic books. They were a quarter apiece back then. A three-dollar allowance which I earned, every penny went a long way back then. (Larry Coots, Pomfret Center, Connecticut)

Notes

Chapter 1

1. See Samuel Merwin, *Rise and Fight Againe,* New York: Albert and Charles Boni, Inc., 1935; hereafter referred to in text as *"RFA."* Samuel Merwin was to Liggett what Boswell was to Johnson, and his book, *Rise and Fight Againe,* was a paean to Liggett. Merwin admitted bias, but his account is essential to an understanding of how Rexall began, and it was essential to the account that follows.

2. Untitled, undated, anonymous manuscript providing detailed descriptions of portions of Rexall history; hereafter referred to in text as "Rexall ms." This manuscript, supplied by Ruth Pohlman, is believed by one Rexall retiree to have been written by a Reed Crain (?). Authorship has not been confirmed by this author.

3. Rexall Store Meeting Bulletin, undated, anonymous; hereafter referred to in text as "Rexall bulletin."

Chapter 3

1. These "PC" references are from personal communications with Rexall retirees. The numbers refer to the identities of the sources, which I have on file. I have promised not to identify these sources, mostly Rexall retirees, without their permission. On request from the reader, I will contact the source to ask permission to supply the identity.

Chapter 4

1. Mickey C. Smith, *Pharmaceutical Marketing: Strategy and Cases,* Binghamton, NY: The Haworth Press, 1991. The updated version of the text is Mickey C. Smith, E. M. "Mick" Kolassa, Greg Perkins, and Bruce Sieker, *Pharmaceutical Marketing: Principles, Environment, and Practice.* Binghamton, NY: The Haworth Press, 2002.

2. *The Rexall Drug Store Family Almanac and Moon Book;* hereafter referred to in text as *"Rexall Almanac."*

Chapter 7

1. Larry Thomas (Ed.), *The Rexall Story,* St. Louis: Terminal Railroad Association of St. Louis Historical and Technical Society, Inc., 2000; hereafter referred to in text as *"Rexall Story."* There is rich technical detail in Thomas's book, and the reader is urged to try to get a copy. For our purposes we must focus on the promotional aspects.

2. For more information on Alice Faye, see Jane L. Elder, *Alice Faye: A Life Beyond the Silver Screen,* Jackson, MS: University Press of Mississippi, 2002; hereafter referred to in text as *"Alice Faye."*

3. This material originally appeared in Mickey Smith's book *Pharmacy and Medicine on the Air,* Metuchen, NJ: Scarecrow Press, 1989; hereafter referred to in text as *"PMA."*

4. Dan Carson at Rexall Square. *Radiogram,* 28(11).

Chapter 8

1. For detailed histories of Walgreens, which I have drawn upon in this chapter, see *Walgreens Celebrating 100 Years As the Pharmacy America Trusts,* Company publication, 2001; hereafter referred to as *100 Years;* and *Drug Store News* 22(15), October 16, 2000, a special edition devoted entirely to the 100th anniversary of Walgreens.

2. Herman and Rick Kogan, *Pharmacist to the Nation: A History of Walgreen Company, America's Leading Drug Store Chain,* Chicago: The Walgreen Company, 1989; hereafter referred to in text as *"History of Walgreen."*

Index

Advertising, 110-111
    magazine, 120-121
    radio, 121-134, 141
    television, 133-134. *See also photo
        section*
Amos 'n' Andy, 121, 131
Aspirin, 91-92

Beattie, Robert, 143
Bergen Drug Company, 39
BismaRex, 62, 106, 110, 114-115
Bowles, John, 29-30, 35, 37, 144, 168
Bowles, Norma, 29-30
Bristol Myers, 10

Cahoon, E. D., 6
Cara Nome, 115, 130
Channel relationships, 83
Chronology, *xx-xxi*
Clerk training, 92-94, 98-104
Crown Drug, 150

Dan Carson's story, 132. *See also photo
        section*
Dart, Justin, 28-29, 33-34, 37-42, 44,
        47, 115, 122-123, 137-148.
        See also photo section
    political activities, 42, 137-138
    and Walgreen, 138
Dart Industries, 38, 45, 149-150
Dear Pardner letters, 12, 17-28, 81, 117
DeMoville, James, 4-6, 73

Distribution, 44, 81, 112
Dockum, Harry, 10. *See also photo
        section*
Duncan Drugs, 165-168. *See also photo
        section*

Equate brand, 33, 57, 68

Federal Trade Commission, 73
Fibber McGee and Molly, 70, 121
Franchises, 105-108, 139-140. *See also
        photo section*

Galvin, Joseph, 12, 36, 138
Gathright-Reed Drug. *See also photo
        section*
Goldfish Promotion, 38. *See also photo
        section*
Guth Chocolate Company, 8, 53

Hazard Rexall Drugs, 165-169. *See
        also photo section*

Jimmy Durante Show, 121, 139

Kentucky, Hazard, 165
Klenzo, 115, 167
Kraft Foods, 53

Letters, customer, 85-91
Liggett, Louis, 3-16, 116-117. *See also*
    photo section
    beginning business, 3-5
    financial problems, 10, 24-25
    honorary degrees, 15
    retirement, 12
Liggett Company formation, 8
Logos. *See photo section*

Mutual Fire Insurance Company, 22

Narcotics, 8
National Association of Retail
    Druggists, 46
National Cigar Stands, 7

One-Cent Sale, 31, 33, 35-36, 45,
    67-80, 82-83, 107-108. *See also*
    photo section
Original stockholders, 5-6
Owl Drug Stores, 10-11
Own Goods, 84

Pepper Pod, 145
Pharmacy education, 163
Phil Harris/Alice Faye Show, 36, 70,
    122-131. *See also photo*
    section
Plenamins, 128
Prescriptions, 63-66, 157-159. *See also*
    photo section
    free, 8
Price, 67-80
Product strategy, 51-66
Production, 52
Promotion, 113-136. *See also photo*
    section
Puretest Products, 53-54

Quality control, 52-53, 60-61

Radio advertising, 121, 134
Rex lawsuit, 21
Rexall
    Ad-Vantages, 54-55, 64, 68-69, 73,
        102-104, 117-120
    Almanac, 58-59, 120
    course on business, 97-98
    Family Druggist, 51, 126-130
    logo. *See photo section*
    Magazine, 8, 104, 120. *See also*
        photo section
    Magic Hour, 70, 121
    name, 6-7
    News, 104, 120
    Parade of Stars, 121
    Reporter, 104
    research, 11, 60-61, 106, 114
    signs, 36, 63. *See also photo section*
    train, 11, 12, 113-116. *See also*
        photo section
Rexall retirees, 27
Rexall Sundown Company, 30, 45, 154
Rexall-logues, 94-97
Riker Drug Company, 8, 62, 66,
    141-142
Ross-Hall, 29-30, 43-47, 150

Saint Louis Plant. *See photo section*
Sales force, 104-105
Saxona, 6
Seamless Rubber Company, 8, 12
Stage play, 74-80
Sterling Products, 10-11, 54
Stock market, 10-12, 23
Super Plenamins, 28, 63, 110, 129, 134,
    151. *See also photo section*

Talking Penny, 70-73
Television advertising, 133-134. *See*
    also photo section

Trailers, 62
Tupperware, 29, 38, 40, 42, 141-142

United Cigar Stores, 8
United Drug Company, 9, 10. *See also photo section*
United Drug Company, Canada, 54

Vander Linden, Howard, 151-152
Vicks Chemical Company, 54

Vinol Club, 4
Vitamin Corporation of America, 141

Walgreen Company, 31, 34, 41, 116, 144-147, 160
  and pharmacy education, 146-147
Wal-Mart, 33, 67-68
War efforts, 8-9, 12, 22, 60-61
Weber, Larry, 152-153
Wholesaling, 112

Order a copy of this book with this form or online at:
http://www.haworthpress.com/store/product.asp?sku=5190

THE REXALL STORY
A History of Genius and Neglect

_____in hardbound at $39.95 (ISBN: 0-7890-2472-1)

_____in softbound at $24.95 (ISBN: 0-7890-2473-X)

Or order online and use special offer code HEC25 in the shopping cart.

COST OF BOOKS_____	☐ **BILL ME LATER:** (Bill-me option is good on US/Canada/Mexico orders only; not good to jobbers, wholesalers, or subscription agencies.)
	☐ Check here if billing address is different from shipping address and attach purchase order and billing address information.
POSTAGE & HANDLING_____ *(US: $4.00 for first book & $1.50 for each additional book)* *(Outside US: $5.00 for first book & $2.00 for each additional book)*	
	Signature_____
SUBTOTAL_____	☐ **PAYMENT ENCLOSED: $_____**
IN CANADA: ADD 7% GST_____	☐ **PLEASE CHARGE TO MY CREDIT CARD.**
STATE TAX_____ *(NY, NJ, OH, MN, CA, IL, IN, & SD residents, add appropriate local sales tax)*	☐ Visa ☐ MasterCard ☐ AmEx ☐ Discover ☐ Diner's Club ☐ Eurocard ☐ JCB
FINAL TOTAL_____ *(If paying in Canadian funds, convert using the current exchange rate, UNESCO coupons welcome)*	Account # _____ Exp. Date_____ Signature_____

Prices in US dollars and subject to change without notice.

NAME_____

INSTITUTION_____

ADDRESS_____

CITY_____

STATE/ZIP_____

COUNTRY_____ COUNTY (NY residents only)_____

TEL_____ FAX_____

E-MAIL_____

May we use your e-mail address for confirmations and other types of information? ☐ Yes ☐ No
We appreciate receiving your e-mail address and fax number. Haworth would like to e-mail or fax special discount offers to you, as a preferred customer. **We will never share, rent, or exchange your e-mail address or fax number.** We regard such actions as an invasion of your privacy.

Order From Your Local Bookstore or Directly From
The Haworth Press, Inc.
10 Alice Street, Binghamton, New York 13904-1580 • USA
TELEPHONE: 1-800-HAWORTH (1-800-429-6784) / Outside US/Canada: (607) 722-5857
FAX: 1-800-895-0582 / Outside US/Canada: (607) 771-0012
E-mailto: orders@haworthpress.com

For orders outside US and Canada, you may wish to order through your local
sales representative, distributor, or bookseller.
For information, see http://haworthpress.com/distributors

(Discounts are available for individual orders in US and Canada only, not booksellers/distributors.)
PLEASE PHOTOCOPY THIS FORM FOR YOUR PERSONAL USE.
http://www.HaworthPress.com   BOF04